Francis K. O. Yuen
Editor

Social Work Practice
with Children and Families
A Family Health Approach

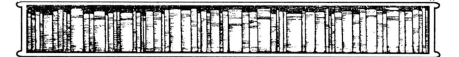

Social Work Practice
with Children and Families
A Family Health Approach

HAWORTH Social Work Practice
with Children and Families
John T. Pardeck, PhD, LCSW
Senior Editor

Family Health Social Work Practice with Children and Families by Francis K. O. Yuen

Homelessness in Rural America: Policy and Practice by Paul A. Rollinson and John T. Pardeck

Handbook for the Treatment of Abused and Neglected Children by Peter Forrest Talley

Titles of Related Interest:

Grandparents As Carers of Children with Disabilities: Facing the Challenges edited by Philip McCallion and Matthew P. Janicki

Family-Centered Services in Residential Treatment: New Approaches for Group Care edited by John Y. Powell

Caring on the Streets: A Study of Detached Youthworkers edited by Jacquelyn K. Thompson

Family Health Social Work Practice: A Knowledge and Skills Casebook by Francis K. O. Yuen, Gregory J. Skibinski, and John T. Pardeck

Social Work Practice with Children and Families
A Family Health Approach

Francis K. O. Yuen
Editor

The Haworth Social Work Practice Press™
An Imprint of The Haworth Press, Inc.
New York • London • Oxford

For more information on this book or to order, visit
http://www.haworthpress.com/store/product.asp?sku=5305

or call 1-800-HAWORTH (800-429-6784) in the United States and Canada
or (607) 722-5857 outside the United States and Canada

or contact orders@HaworthPress.com

Published by

The Haworth Social Work Practice Press™, an imprint of The Haworth Press, Inc., 10 Alice Street,
Binghamton, NY 13904-1580.

PUBLISHER'S NOTE
Identities and circumstances of individuals discussed in this book have been changed to protect
confidentiality.

Cover design by Marylouise E. Doyle.

Library of Congress Cataloging-in-Publication Data

Social work practice with children and families : a family health approach / Francis K. O. Yuen,
editor.
        p.   cm.
     Includes bibliographical references and index.
     ISBN 0-7890-1795-4 (hard : alk. paper)—ISBN 0-7890-1796-2 (soft : alk. paper)
     1. Family social work. 2. Social work with children. 3. Family—Health and hygiene. I. Yuen,
Francis K. O. II. Series.
HV697.S58 2005
362.7—dc22
                                                                              2004014890

To my mother,
Mrs. Wai Sheung Wong-Yuen

CONTENTS

ABOUT THE EDITOR

Francis K. O. Yuen, DSW, ACSW, is a Professor in the Division of Social Work at California State University in Sacramento. He is widely published in the areas of family health social work practice, disability, grant writing, program planning and evaluation, substance abuse, international social work, and services to refugees and immigrants. He is a member of several editorial boards, including those of the *Journal of Social Work in Disability & Rehabilitation* and the *Journal of Ethnic & Cultural Diversity in Social Work*. He has authored and edited many books, including several for The Haworth Press, Inc., such as *Family Health Social Work Practice: A Knowledge and Skills Casebook* (2003), *International Perspectives on Disability Services: The Same But Different* (2004), and the upcoming *Disability and Social Work Education: Practice and Policy Issues*. His interests in family health practice involve theoretical foundation, management and evaluation, community practice, and intervention skills.

CONTRIBUTORS

Chrystal C. Ramirez Barranti, PhD, MSW, is an assistant professor for the Division of Social Work at California State University, Sacramento. She has published in the areas of grandparenthood, aging and families, lesbian families, multicultural communications, Latina/Latino families, and Mexican migrant farmworking families. Her interests are in social work practice with elders and with Mexican immigrant families.

Joyce Burris, PhD, MSW, is a professor for the Division of Social Work at California State University, Sacramento. She teaches death and dying, human behavior in the social environment, and advanced policy courses. Her research interests include constructivism, aging, death and loss, and child development.

George E. Connor, PhD, is an associate professor of political science at Southwest Missouri State University. He is an eclectic scholar whose interests range from Congress to biblical criticism. These interests include applying concepts of political culture to educational and legal institutions.

Susan C. Dollar, PhD, LCSW, is an assistant professor in the School of Social Work, Southwest Missouri State University. Her interests in family health focus on rural health services and prevention education, particularly with Latinas/Latinos and those affected by HIV/AIDS.

Susan Talamantes Eggman, PhD, MSW, is an assistant professor for the Division of Social Work at California State University, Sacramento. Her practice has been in medical social work, and she has developed a student internship program in a nonprofit organization serving the working poor and homeless.

John L. Erlich, MSW, ACSW, ABD, is a professor in the Division of Social Work, California State University, Sacramento. He has published extensively in the areas of community intervention and community organizing, planning, and diversity. He is co-author of *Strategies of Community Intervention, Community Organizing in a Diverse Society,* and *Tactics and Techniques of Community Intervention.*

Robin Kennedy, PhD, MSW, is an assistant professor at California State University, Sacramento, where she teaches social work practice, human behavior in the social environment, and medical social work. Her research interests include gay and lesbian family issues, medical social work, and forensic social work.

Nicole Nicotera, PhD, MSW, is an assistant professor for the Graduate School of Social Work at the University of Denver. She has extensive social work practice experience with children and families in community mental health and public school settings. Her research interests include the contextual effects of neighborhoods on children and families and the amplification of neighborhood as a component for assessment and intervention in direct social work practice.

Ute C. Orgassa, PhD, Dipl. Soz. Paed., received her social work training both in Germany and in the United States. She has worked with families with children with disabilities and has published on this topic as well. Her research interests include the impacts of disabilities and the competence of families and individuals in meeting these changes. She currently resides in Pasadena, California.

John T. Pardeck, PhD, LCSW, was a professor for the School of Social Work at Southwest Missouri State University and was a University Research Fellow. He published many books and numerous articles in academic and professional journals. He was the senior editor for the *Journal of Social Work in Disability & Rehabilitation.* His areas of interest in family health included theory building, social policy, and disability issues. His latest publications included *Social Work After the Americans with Disabilities Act: New Challenges and Opportunities for Social Service Professionals, Family Health Social Work Practice: A Macro Level Approach,* and *Family Health Social Work Practice: A Knowledge and Skills Casebook.* Leaving behind a legacy of scholarship and social justice, Dr. Pardeck passed away in November 2004.

Christine A. Price, PhD, is an assistant professor and extension state gerontology specialist in the Department of Human Development and Family Science at The Ohio State University. Her programming interests include grandparents raising grandchildren, end-of-life issues, aging families, and universal design to promote aging in place. She has multiple research publications pertaining to women's adult development, specifically women's retirement.

Gregory J. Skibinski, PhD, ACSW, is a professor for the School of Social Work at Southwest Missouri State University and former director of the master of social work (MSW) program. He has many publications in the areas of child sexual abuse, social work practice, and program evaluation. His interests in family health include intervention strategies, child maltreatment, research, and health. His latest book publication is *Family Health Social Work Practice: A Knowledge and Skills Casebook.*

Susan A. Taylor, PhD, MSW, is an associate professor in the Division of Social Work at California State University, Sacramento. She previously taught health policy at Saint Louis University and has also taught child welfare policy and administration. Her research, teaching, and professional interests include family and children's policy development, implementation, and planning in governmental and nongovernmental settings.

Foreword

I am pleased to write this foreword for my friend and colleague, Francis Yuen, who is a fellow professor of social work at California State University, Sacramento, where I have taught for thirty years.

Dr. Yuen's editorship of *Social Work Practice with Children and Families: A Family Health Approach* is a continuing indicator of his many achievements. He has edited and/or co-authored many texts on family health, grant writing and program evaluation, violent youth, teenage pregnancy and parenthood, children with emotional and behavioral difficulties, and disability services, and he has written numerous journal articles and book chapters.

The focus of this book is on children and families. Beginning with a conceptual understanding of family health social work practice, Dr. Yuen distinguishes various approaches for defining and understanding health issues and urges readers to change their perspectives on health and family practice. Contributors address family health practice interventions as well as policy, programs, and emerging family themes, and they include case studies and examples.

Regarding practice interventions, Skibinski and Connor focus on child sexual abuse examination and treatment processes, highlight the importance of diversion programs, and suggest helpful child sexual abuse litigation strategies. Pardeck introduces the use of bibliotherapy when working with children of divorced parents and offers practical steps to match appropriate books with specific problems. Dollar addresses adaptive strategies for assisting rural families living with HIV/AIDS and discusses high-risk groups, poverty, and the multiple impacts and stressors on, as well as family and community interventions for, this emerging and neglected population. Orgassa contributes on the topic of families with children with disabilities and utilizes a crisis intervention helping model that reflects family health care services. Burris centers on children's reactions to loss in terms of grief and coping, offers practical ways of helping, and discusses developmental issues involved in the process. Ramirez Barranti explores the personal characteristics of Mexican migrant and seasonal farmworking families, particularly the biopsychosocial dimensions and life experiences of this group.

Addressing policy and program concerns, Price highlights an increasingly visible family pattern of grandparents as parents and helps readers understand the concerns of custodial grandparents. She underlines psychosocial challenges, racial and ethnic considerations, problem behaviors of grandchildren, and relationship issues with adult children. Kennedy writes about lesbian and gay families and comments on legal inequities, such as custody laws, health insurance, tax laws, medical care, and estate planning. She also focuses on the current state of gay and lesbian families, legal interventions, health care, and the developmental stages of these families. Taylor analyzes the child welfare and foster care policies affecting family health and well-being, pointing out service differentiation, policies of contradictory care, child welfare services, and the need for child health care services. Eggman portrays the health care needs of homeless women with children, discussing demographics, historical events, poverty and homelessness, and previous health care policies for homeless families. She revisits the issues of health and health care for homeless families and offers an interesting model of family health care for this population. Nicotera opens up the neighborhood as a resource for family health care practice, discusses understanding the neighborhood as a habitat and niche, and reviews literature from the adult's and child's worldviews. She suggests that the neighborhood is an appropriate resource for understanding assessment and intervention. Finally, Erlich examines family health and community practice and focuses on decent housing, safe streets, adequate transportation, day care, and recreation. His paradigm revolves around two programs: PREPARE (Problems, Reality, Establish, People, Assess, Risks, Evaluate) and IMAGINE (Idea, Muster, Assets, Goals, Implement, Neutralize, Evaluate).

This text, *Social Work Practice with Children and Families,* along with the companion volume, *Family Health Social Work Practice: A Knowledge and Skills Casebook* (The Haworth Social Work Practice Press, 2003), combine to offer the best practice texts available for the emerging social work advanced curriculum on family health in the United States. Social work education programs interested in mounting family health specializations now have the necessary literary resources. The Haworth Press is to be commended for publishing in this new and emerging subject. Dr. Yuen is to be congratulated on his work in this area and is considered a pioneer in family health social work as a field of study.

Doman Lum, PhD, ThD
Professor Emeritus of Social Work
California State University, Sacramento

Acknowledgments

"Dedication to professional competency and academic excellence" accurately describes the commitment and efforts of the chapter contributors for this book. Behind these contributors are their spouses, partners, children, and families whose understanding and support have made their professional pursuits possible. For this important reason, I would like to express my sincere appreciation.

John T. Pardeck, senior editor for The Haworth Press Social Work Practice with Children and Families series was an invaluable advisor and confidant. His insight into family health social work practice and his encouragement were instrumental to the completion of this book project. Greg Skibinski, an outstanding social work educator and a great friend, completed his chapter in the ICU at a hospital. I commend Greg and admire his dedication. Terry Brown's detailed and expert editorial support to the last minute is much appreciated.

I am grateful for the support, patience, flexibility, and expertise of the staff at The Haworth Press. I am also in debt to my students for their valuable critiques, insights, encouragement, and inspiration.

Chapter 1

Family Health Social Work Practice and Change

Francis K. O. Yuen

Family health social work practice emphasizes the attainment of the holistic well-being of a family system and its members. Family health is "manifested by the development of, and continuous interaction among, the economic, physical, mental, emotional, social, cultural, and spiritual dimensions of the family that results in its holistic well-being as well as that of its members" (Yuen and Skibinski, 2003, p. 205).

FAMILY HEALTH SOCIAL WORK PRACTICE

Family is defined as a system of two or more interacting persons who are either related by ties of marriage, birth, or adoption, or who have chosen to commit themselves in unity for the common purpose of promoting the physical, mental, emotional, social, economic, cultural, and spiritual growth and development of the unit and each of its members (Pardeck and Yuen, 1999). Family can be further conceptualized by its interrelated dimensions of nature, structure, and function (Pardeck and Yuen, 1997; Pardeck et al., 1998).

"The nature of a family is its essential characteristics and qualities. . . . It is characterized by its unconditional concerns or commitment for the total well-being of its members and itself" (Yuen and Skibinski, 2003, p. 204). It is not uncommon to see parents put their children's welfare and desires ahead of their own. They may even sacrifice everything they have, including their lives, to protect or sup-

1

port their young ones. These unconditional concerns and commitments sharply distinguish a family from other intimate social groups.

The structure of a family refers to the composition and the transactional patterns among the family members. The family structure establishes the roles, norms, and patterns of interaction among its members. There are male-headed, heterosexual, two-parent families with children. There are also female-headed single-parent families or families of gay parents and their children. An increasing number of grandparents are raising their grandchildren. Within each of these families, different transactional patterns affect and dictate the behaviors of the family members.

Family functions comprise "the activities necessary for realizing the family's common purpose. . . . The functions of a family are intricately tied to the needs of the family" (Yuen and Skibinski, 2003, p. 204). These activities attend to the fulfillment of the physical, mental, social, economic, spiritual, and cultural growth of the family unit and its members. Not all families have the capacities or the needs to carry out all of these functions. These capacities are affected by social, political, and economic conditions of society at the time. The extent to which a family is capable of fulfilling all or a selected few of these functions is directly correlated to the well-being of the family.

The concept of health for family health practice is more than the absence of physical or mental diseases; it is about the holistic state of "being connected in a fulfilling way with the natural and human world" (Pardeck et al., 1998, p. 28). Yuen and Pardeck (1999) explain the differences among the disease, illness, sickness, and family health models (see Table 1.1).

The disease model is based on a biomedical approach, in which professionals or experts make an objective diagnosis and identify one's pathological symptoms. The presence of symptoms or the expert's diagnosis determines one's state of health. Intervention or change strategies include enlisting the help of experts or professionals to overcome symptoms and their causes.

The illness model relies on subjective and personal perceptions. These personal assertions, however, need to be confirmed by a professional. One is ill as long as the individual and the experts psychologically believe the person is ill. Health is therefore personal and subjective. A cancer survivor may consider herself living a fulfilling and healthy life, while a hypochondriac may believe he is ill and suf-

TABLE 1.1. Approaches for defining and understanding health.

	Disease model	Illness	Sickness model	Family health perspective
Basis	Biomedical	Psychological	Sociological	Biopsychosocial/ecological
Orientation	Pathological symptoms	Subjective perception	Socially constructed	Ecological and family systems
Assessment and intervention	Professional objective diagnosis of symptoms	Professional evaluations and understanding of one's self-constructed conditions	Professional assessments of psychosocial environment	Professional interventions based on the dynamics of people's subjective perspectives and changing their social environment

Source: From Yuen, F. and Pardeck, J. (1999). A family health approach to social work practice. In J. T. Pardeck and F. K. O. Yuen (Eds.), *Family health: A holistic approach to social work practice* (p. 4). Westport, CT: Auburn House.

fering from physical ailments. The word *ill* in the illness model has a specific meaning, which is different from its general usage, such as when describing mental illness or someone who is physically ill.

In the sickness model, sickness is a sociological construct in which individuals exhibit certain socially unacceptable behaviors for which they may be considered sick. Beyond physical or mental conditions, sickness implies the application of and judgment by social or moral standards. The degree of adherence to, deviation from, or attainment of socially desirable standards determines one's state of health. This construct is affected by the ever-evolving social and cultural norms. Alcoholics' drinking habits and their associated problems cause certain people to consider alcoholics as being sick. The changing view on alcoholism, from being caused by personal character deficits (sickness) to recognizing it as a medical condition (disease), addresses some of the social stigmas, and allows many who might otherwise avoid it to seek treatment.

Figure 1.1 summarizes and displays the theoretical orientations of family health social work practice (Yuen, 2003, p. 20). It represents the integration and application of a set of related theories, perspectives, and practice principles that inform the family health approach. They include systems theory, ecological perspectives, social constructionist perspectives, human diversity considerations, individual and family developmental theories, and theories on family interventions. The family health approach supports interdisciplinary collaborations and promotes the eclectic use of a collection of appropriate intervention modalities. It also proposes a list of beginning practice approaches and skills (Pardeck et al., 1998):

1. Conduct developmental assessment that includes biopsychosocial and cultural assessments of the individual, family, and social network to set the foundation for proper interventions.
2. Access and link both formal and informal resources.
3. Provide supportive and empathetic intervention that builds on professional relationships and appreciates diversity.
4. Use confrontative strategies within an empowerment framework.

5. Advocate for the client to promote social justice and to secure appropriate services.
6. Facilitate the empowerment of the client based on strength perspectives.
7. Utilize psychoeducation and social learning strategies to augment therapeutic and other interventions for change.
8. Recognize the level of prevention (primary, secondary, and tertiary) and readiness for change.
9. Use the family unit as a change agent since it is a particularly potent force for change. Assess issues such as family communication, power dynamics, cohesion, and reality constructions.

The social work profession believes in change. Social workers trust that clients have the capacities to make change. In many situations, clients' environments may be the targets for improvement. Social workers see their roles to be the change agents for these processes. These may be micro- (individual), mezzo- (group), or macro-level (community and organization) changes that affect a target population's knowledge, attitude, and behavior. Without this belief in people and their ability as well as the possibility to invoke change, social work practice would become merely a time-wasting and meaningless exercise of human interactions.

Why do people want to change? How can family health social workers help facilitate the change? Clients or service recipients come to social workers' attention voluntarily or involuntarily. Some are highly motivated, whereas others are reluctant or unsure about their involvement and the necessity for change. Compton and Galaway (1998) describe people who seek social work assistance as individuals who are encountering life conditions that have overwhelmed them and their means of solution. Ideally, after a thorough biopsychosocial and cultural assessment, a family health social worker will develop and implement appropriate intervention plans and actions for change. In some environments, particularly in crisis situations, however, the likelihood of a thorough assessment is limited. Nevertheless, family health social workers should strive to understand clients' reasons and needs for change, engage clients in working for change, and take aim at the outcomes of change.

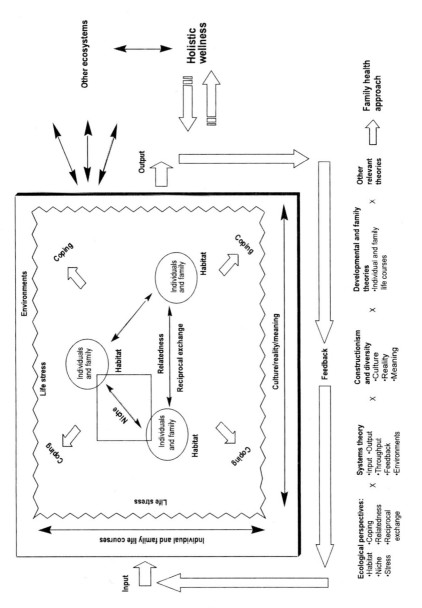

FIGURE 1.1. Theoretical orientations of a family health approach.

REASONS AN NEEDS FOR CHANGE

Social workers use empat tic understanding and critical thinking skills to help them learn and c plain a client's situation within the client's own context and envi onment. Professional training in areas such as human behavior and social environment, human diversity, and social policy is designed to develop a capacity for understanding without being judgmental. Informed by this knowledge and understanding, social workers purposely complete a biopsychosocial assessment for their clients during the initial contacts. The aim is to understand the clients and their situations in a manner that is culturally, developmentally, socially, and spiritually appropriate. It is also important to assess clients' unique concerns, strengths, and challenges. Based on this assessment, social workers work with clients to formulate the agreed-upon change and provide them with appropriate support.

Isaac Newton discovered the grand theories of motion for physics. His first law of motion states that an object at rest will remain at rest and an object in motion will continue in motion at the same speed unless acted upon by an external force. We conduct our lives in set ways, believing there is no need for change. The inertia of disinclining to change is strong, and the desire to change is minimal. This property of matter remains unchanged until another force pushes the object to change its course.

Clients who come to social workers for assistance are usually dealing with life situations that demand change. Along with external forces, there are internal and inherent desires and capacity within a person to change for the better. It is difficult to expect a mother with family management problems to go eagerly to a parenting class in between her two part-time jobs and within her chaotic family situations. It may be a court order or a social worker's recommendation that is the initial force that gets her to participate in the class. Her own desires to become a better parent and improve her family life may be as much if not more important motivation for her participation in the class than the external pressure. Social workers play a key role in encouraging and promoting their clients' realizations, desires, and capacities for change. Subsequent to a client's decision to change, social workers have the responsibility to help clients identify ways they can attain that change.

Beisser (1970) describes Frederick Perls's, the founder of Gestalt therapy, views on the theory of change. Perls believed that "change occurs when one becomes what he is, not when he tries to become what he is not" (Beisser, 1970). Perls maintained that clients who seek change experience conflicts between who they are and who they should be. He further believed that changes could only happen after the client accepts himself or herself as who he or she is. It is the experience of the client at that moment of truth that provides the foundation for the client to move forward and to change. Service providers with different theoretical orientations have different views on why and how people change. Behaviorists attempt to change behaviors through behavioral modifications. Psychoanalytic therapists try to identify insights that lead to change.

Certainly, in many social work practice situations, clients do not come to receive service because they want to but because they have to. Some may come voluntarily but without a clear idea of why they are there. Rooney (1992) describes these people as clients who are being forced or coerced into a relationship in which they feel disadvantaged. These clients have been called "hostile, resistant, reluctant, unmotivated, dysfunctional, hard-to-reach, and multi-problem" (p. 7). These terms "cast a pejorative light on the presumed client characteristics rather than on the nature of the contact between client and practitioner" (p. 7). Rooney goes on to lay out legal, ethical, and effective practice strategies for working with involuntary clients.

What is a need? Meyers (1985) states Bradshaw's (1977) four types of needs for social work practice (Yuen and Terao, 2003): normative, felt, expressed, and comparative. Normative needs are conditions that are below the established standard. Clients living below the poverty line and in neighborhoods with higher-than-average unemployment rates are in situations that need change. Felt needs are individual desires and standards that are particular to certain people. Many older adults who live alone prefer to stay in their own homes while maintaining regular social contacts with others. Ethnic clients may wish to work with social workers who are culturally and linguistically appropriate to the clients' backgrounds. Expressed needs are documented or explicitly articulated demands. A town hall meeting on the public safety of a community, a needs-assessment survey of local concerns about the recent increase of hate crimes, or a waiting list of people who want mental health counseling are all examples of expressed needs that lead to changes. Comparative needs are conditions that affect certain populations more than others. Teenage mothers in alternative schools experience a higher level of stress than their peers attending traditional high schools. Socially isolated older adults, in comparison to other older adults who live with families, may have a greater need for services that allow them to become more socially connected and therefore enjoy a more successful aging. Teenage mothers may need additional personal and academic support to help them to complete school and care for themselves and their children.

There are many ways to answer the question "Why change?" Simply, people want answers that allow them to see that a particular cause (e.g., reason, need) directly explains a particular change (e.g., effect, result). However, in most social work practice situations, the clear-cut answer of causation to the question "why" is not easy to obtain. Often, too many interrelated factors or conditions led to the presence of the client's current situation.

A causal relation can be established only in the presence of a "list of conditions which together are considered necessary and sufficient to explain the occurrence of the phenomenon in question" (Chafetz, 1978, p. 22). Chafetz further explains that "a necessary explanation is one in which the elements listed must be present to bring about the result in question" (p. 22). The presence of clouds is necessary for rainfall to occur, but a cloud alone is not enough to cause rain. It is not possible to have rain under a clear blue sky, but it is possible to have a cloudy day with no rain in sight. "A sufficient explanation is one in which the elements listed will always bring about the result in question" (Chafetz, 1978, p. 22). A spoonful of cyanide is enough to kill a person if untreated. The presence of enough cyanide in a person's body can bring about death. Cyanide is a sufficient cause for death, but it is not necessary for anyone to have cyanide in order to die. A cloud is a necessary but not sufficient condition for rainfall just as cyanide is a sufficient but not necessary condition for death. Nevertheless, both are important and key contributing factors that bring about the results in question.

Very often social work practice can be working with only key contributing factors rather than absolute root causes. These contributing factors are associated or correlated to the clients' current conditions. By making changes to the contributing factors, and with the ultimate outcomes in mind, social workers attempt to increase the likelihood of attaining the desirable results and eliminating the undesirable results.

Medical doctors, supported by rigorous scientific testing and clinical studies, can pinpoint a particular virus, bacteria, or biological agent that causes a particular disease. Specific medical interventions are therefore used to eliminate or control the cause of the disease in the patient. Unlike medical doctors, social workers cannot deal with causes of issues as if they were viruses or bacteria. They do not know the exact causes for clients' situations and do not have "magic pills" to cure the problem. Similar to medical professionals, however, social workers work with individuals, families, and communities to address issues and factors that affect their health and well-being.

In using the ecosystem approach to understand and explain clients and their situations, social workers also employ the use of "functional explanation." Systems theory asserts that when a change occurs in one part of the client system it also brings about functional change or response from other parts of the system. Functional explanation is different from necessary and sufficient explanation in many respects. Among them, functional explanation does not assume time sequence. "Often, various elements change simultaneously or, when they change sequentially, any one can precede any other and, in fact, succeed it as well" (Chafetz, 1978, p. 25). A biopsychosocial assessment is commonly conducted at the beginning of a social work intervention. It provides the social worker some possible functional explanations of the client's situation.

Different practice models or theories have different assessment focuses and procedures (e.g., the goal of structural family therapy assessment is to understand what has been maintaining the symptoms). Practice settings also dictate the orientations of such assessment (e.g., mental status examination for mental health agencies). Using various established outlines and procedures (e.g., ecomap and genogram), social workers develop a relatively comprehensive and ongoing understanding of the clients' psychosocial, cultural, economic, and spiritual conditions and needs. Through this assessment, social workers identify key issues for intervention and develop clinical impressions or theories about the clients and their situations. Bisman (1999) refers to this impression or working theory as the worker's "case theory," developed to form "the foundation for selection of intervention strategies and methods to achieve change" (p. 240). With the attainment of the family's holistic well-being in mind, family health social workers are to find the proper point of entry into the clients' world, locate clients' urgent or prime concerns, identify key contributing factors, and work with clients to employ the most appropriate and theory-informed intervention to generate goal-oriented change.

WORKING FOR CHANGE
AND OUTCOMES OF CHANGE

If social work practice were stopped at assessing and understanding clients' concerns, it would do no more than tell the clients what they already knew except in some organized jargons. This offers no practical helps to the clients. It is the formulation of intervention plans and the implementation of such interventions that bring about the agreed-upon changes to improve clients' situation. Payne (1997, p. 39) describes three types of social work theories: "theories of what social work is" (e.g., purpose of welfare, welfare state, feminism), "theories of how to do social work" (e.g., case work, family therapy, and group work), and "theories of the client world" (e.g., family, personality, human behavior and social environment, and race). Working for changes and for outcomes is about "how to do social work," the process that brings about the change.

Family therapy as one of the many ways to address the needs of a family in stress has evolved over the past decades into many theories and models. It has also become an independent field of study. Social workers have played a vital role in pioneering as well as developing and applying family therapy. The following are some of the major models and their key figures:

- Strategic therapy (Jay Haley, Don Jackson, and Virginia Satir)
- Structural family therapy (Salvador Minuchin)
- Humanistic and communication approaches (Virginia Satir and Carl Whitaker)
- Solution-focused brief therapy (Steve de Shazer and Insoo Kim Berg)
- Behavioral and cognitive-behavioral family therapy (Ivan Pavlov, B. F. Skinner, Albert Bandura, Albert Ellis, and Aaron Beck)

- Social construction/postmodernism therapy (Kenneth Gergen, Harlene Anderson)
- Narrative family therapy (Harry Goolishian, Michael White, and David Epston)
- Intergenerational family therapy (Murray Bowen)
- Psychoeducational family therapy (Carol Anderson)
- Family preservation practice (Betty Blythe and Bernice Weissbourd)

Snyder (1992) asserts that although approaches for family therapy "may differ in emphasis, they share theoretical basis and share many of the same techniques and interventions. All see the family as a system developing over an intergenerational life cycle" (p. 30). She further identifies the general goals and techniques of family therapies (pp. 27-30):

1. Family therapy focuses on changes in people's here-and-now interactions with others. It is not concerned with what caused a problem but with what seems to maintain it.
2. Family therapy is less reliant on insight than are psychodynamic models.
3. Reframing means relabeling or otherwise redefining behaviors or situations and/or changing the context presented. It is used to expand the family members' views or to reorient them.
4. Teaching communication skills is necessary, and changing the patterns of family communications is achieved by blocking certain interactions and facilitating others.
5. The cost and benefits of problem behaviors should be explored with family.
6. The uses of metaphor help family members grasp the meaning, understand a problem, and envision alternative outcomes. It is also used to plant ideas.
7. Family sculpting creates powerful images that allow family members to gain new understanding of how other members experience them. An example is to ask family members to physically rearrange themselves in ways that illustrate how they perceive themselves in relation to one another.
8. The use of directing activities, such as contracting, homework assignment, skills development, and modeling, is suggested.

The technology of family therapy is often incorporated in social work practice with families. It is utilized under the broad and inclusive mission of the social work profession within the ecosystem framework and is guided by principles such as empowerment, advocacy, social justice, and human diversity. Family health social work practice employs family theories and family therapy models as part of its service delivery technologies to meet the clients' service needs.

Reid (2002) reviews the trends and movements of the knowledge of direct social work practice. Social work practice models were dominated by psychoanalytic methods during the post–World War II period. In the 1950s and 1960s, alternative approaches such as "family systems, behavioral, transactional, gestalt, existential, reality, and cognitive" approaches emerged (p. 8). In the 1970s, many new practice movements came into view. Among them were "the generalist, ecosystems, ecological perspective, strengths perspective, feminist practice, empowerment, task-centered, psychoeducational, solution-focused, multicultural, narrative, family preservation, and empirical practice movements" (p. 8). The influx and rise of these new frameworks reflected the diversity of and openness to new ideas for social work practice. Many attempted to provide integrative practice models that incorporate many theoretical frameworks.

Payne (1997) provides detailed reviews of the development of various social work practice theories and their effects on social work practice. The psychodynamic approach (Hamilton, 1950; Richmond, 1917) is influenced by Sigmund Freud's views on development, personality, and his psychoanalytic approach to treatment. It forms the early social work practice approach that focuses on personality, pathology, and clients' insight. Woods and Hollis's psychosocial approach (1990), although having a strong root in psychodynamic theory, emphasizes the idea of "person-in-situation." It aims to combine a client's internal strength with resources in the environment to improve both personal and interpersonal functioning. This approach begins with diagnostic understanding in which worker and client identify problem areas and relevant personality characteristics. Together they choose short- and long-term treatment objectives, which guide the decisions on the selection of treatment procedures.

Perlman (1957) developed the problem-solving social casework approach that examines the "4 Ps": person, problem, place, and process. "The person with whom work is done, the problem presented, the place where work is done, and the work process . . . The focus is how one's ego manages outside relationship" (Payne, 1997, p. 87). In this model, both the client's presenting problems and difficulties in the environment are addressed. Clients seek help because they have failed in their capacity to solve problems. They need assistance in increasing their coping capacity and overcoming barriers. Perlman's works lead the way for many problem-solving approaches, including the crisis-intervention and task-centered approaches in social work practice. Perlman's problem-solving approach, however, is less concerned about task and more "concerned with seeing human life as a process of resolving life issues" (Payne, 1997, p. 119).

Crisis intervention (Caplan, 1965; Parad, 1965) is based on psychodynamic ego psychology and focuses on people's emotional responses to crises. It uses practical tasks to help people readjust and interrupt events that disrupt normal functioning. The task-centered approach (Reid and Epstein, 1972) is not based on any particular psychological or sociological theories but aims to be integrative and eclectic. It focuses on practical tasks that improve people's capacities to deal with life difficulties in a pragmatic manner with defined goals, tasks, and time limits. This approach is not concerned with the underlying causes of people's problems but focuses instead on more of people's abilities and performance in exposing and addressing the problem.

Family has always been a key component and focus for social work practice models. For example, Carter and McGoldrick (1999), two longtime social workers and family therapists, developed the family life cycle perspective in working with diverse families. Kilpatrick and Holland (1999) proposed to understand and work with families according to their various levels of need. Franklin and Jordan (1999) promoted a brief therapy approach within the context of social work practice with different family therapy models and multilevel intervention approaches. Janzen and Harris (1997) integrated different family intervention approaches and provided a family treatment framework for social workers.

Increasingly, case management has become a major professional function for social workers. Case management attempts to assist clients in receiving the most appropriate services in a coordinated and timely manner to bring about the desirable change. Rothman and Sager (1998) proposed a new social work practice paradigm—the comprehensive psychological enhancement approach—for integrated case-management practice. Walsh (2000) discusses different case-management approaches in mental health practice and supported the application of a clinical case-management approach. Walsh described that case-management services can range from basic skills training for preventing relapse to proactive skills development for independent living to strength-based brokering of services to promote client's success. Having a case manager who intimately knows the client's concerns and needs can also play a more direct and therapeutic role in promoting change. This clinical approach of case management requires the worker to engage in psychotherapeutic intervention, brokering of service, crisis intervention, and consultation.

Along with working with the individuals, family health social work practice intervenes in one's mezzo- and macroenvironments to create opportunities for change and development. Services to families are often augmented by promoting changes in neighborhood, community, organization, and social policies at both local and national levels. Family health social workers should be prepared to assume the roles of agency administrators, grant and program developers, community organizers, social planners, legislators, labor organizers, group workers, and many other responsibilities.

Change is a dominant and constant feature of social workers' and clients' lives. Family health social workers as change agents employ different service delivery technologies to help clients develop their own theories of change and achieve the agreed-upon outcomes or results. The Annie E. Casey Foundation (2003) defines theory of change as "a clear expression of the apparent relationships between actions and hoped-for results. It provides an explanation of the reasons why certain strategies are being used and how and in what sequence those strategies will achieve the desired change" (Annie E. Casey Foundation, 2003). This source further lists key elements of the theory of change for a complex community initiative. First, it must have an outcome framework that includes achievable early, immediate, and long-term outcomes. Second, it should include a list of well-founded assumptions that may be about human behaviors, resources, and demographic or economic context. Third, it should identify interventions and their implementation details that would bring about the planned outcomes. As mentioned previously, Bisman (1999) discusses the formulation of a social worker's clinical impression of the client and refers to it as the worker's "case theory." It is a working framework for the attainment of the desirable results of the worker's intervention.

Yuen and Terao (2003) distinguished the various types of intended results of service interventions, namely goals and objectives. "Goals are long-term destinations that are general. They are not necessarily measurable or achievable in the short run" (p. 29). Netting, Kettner, and McMurtry (1993) described goals as "statement(s) of hopes and expectations" (p. 242). Improving clients' quality of life or achieving overall well-being are examples of goals. An objective, on the other hand, "is a statement of measurable and directional change for a specific population in a specific time period" (Yuen and Terao, 2003, p. 9).

Generally, objectives can be further grouped into process objectives, outcome objectives, and impact objectives. A process objective describes "what activities are to be carried out to achieve the planned results" (Yuen and Terao, 2003, p. 9). It is a bean-counting and procedural-oriented objective that tells what will be done or what is expected to happen. Objectives are also referred to as output or accomplishments. For example:

- Fifteen clients will attend the weekly parenting training class.
- The Meals on Wheels program will serve 600 homebound older adults in the next three months.
- The client will record the number of arguments she has with her parents.
- The social worker will explore the client's family history of mental illness.

An outcome objective "focus(es) on the result of the interventions" (Yuen and Terao, 2003, p. 9). It asks about how well the interventions perform and how successful the changes are that result. It questions, What difference, if any, does the intervention make? The following are examples of outcome objectives:

- The client will report a diminishing of depressive mood to no more than three times per week.
- The client will significantly decrease any impulsive reactions to conflictual situations at home.

- At the end of the service period, the client will reunite with her two children who are now in foster care.
- Eighty percent of the participating youth will develop a negative attitude toward tobacco use.

Impact is "the collective and accumulative results of the intervention. Impact objectives aim to answer the question of 'so what?'" (Yuen and Terao, 2003, p. 9). An impact objective describes the desirable end results of the intervention. It is the summary effect that transcends individual interventions. Because impact is not immediate, sometimes it may not be seen within the period of the intervention. For example:

- The Campbell neighborhood will become a safer and more caring community in which children are unlikely to be approached by drug dealers or affected by gang violence.
- The client and his family will have sufficient understanding of his illness and how it can be managed with the help of a home nurse to allow him to stay with his family instead of being placed into an institution.
- Sixty percent of the participating teenage mothers will remain in school to complete their high school education.
- The client will regain her sense of self-worth.

Although fine distinctions can be made among these different types of objectives, no clear line exists that can conclusively determine a process objective from an outcome objective. They are not mutually exclusive. Objectives are contextual. They are determined by the design of the intervention and are relative to the other related objectives. Attending therapy sessions can be a process objective; it may also be an outcome objective. After many attempts (process objective), the reluctant client is finally convinced to attend the sessions (outcome objective). By attending at least 75 percent of the planned sessions (process objective), the client will be able to identify and verbalize his or her irrational beliefs (outcome objective), and understand that he or she can resume normal family and social lives (impact).

Service results can be classified in many ways. They are sometimes referred to generally as outcomes or goals. Many call them short-term and long-term objectives or immediate and long-term outcomes. Others may see them as outputs and outcomes. The choices of names reflect the use of different underlining theories and definitions. No matter how they are titled, they represent the destinations and directions of the service interventions. There are many steps, setbacks, and achievements that one may encounter along the way to attaining the holistic well-being of a family and its members.

A Chinese folktale tells about a man who set out to remove a mountain from in front of his house. Everyone in the village called him a fool. His ambition and commitment, however, set an example for those who want to make change not only through words but also actions. Saint Francis of Assisi reportedly said, "Start by doing what's necessary, then do what's possible, and suddenly you are doing the impossible." Social workers are change agents. Sometimes, changes do not come easily. It is, however, by embarking on carrying away small stones that the removal of a mountain begins.

REFERENCES

Annie E. Casey Foundation (2003). Introduction to the theory of change. Topic paper for Making Connections: A neighborhood transformation family development initiative. Available online at: <www.aecf.org/initiatives/mc/llp/llp_docs/theory_of_changespreads2.pdf>.

Beisser, A. (1970). Paradoxical theory of change. Available online at: <www.gestalt.org/arnie.htm>.

Bisman, C. (1999). Social work assessment: Case theory construction. *Family in Society: The Journal of Contemporary Human Services, 80*(3), 240-247.

Bradshaw, J. (1977). The concept of social need. In N. Gilbert and H. Specht (Eds.), *Planning for social welfare: Issues, tasks, and models* (pp. 290-296). Englewood Cliffs, NJ: Prentice Hall.

Caplan, G. (1965). *Principles of preventive psychiatry*. London: Tavistock.

Carter, B. and McGoldrick, M. (Eds.) (1999). *The expanded family life cycle: Individual, family, and social perspective,* Third edition. Needham Heights, MA: Allyn & Bacon.

Chafetz, J. A. (1978). *A primer on the construction and testing of theories in sociology*. Itasca, IL: F. E. Peacock.

Compton, B. and Galaway, B. (1998). *Social work process,* Sixth edition. Pacific Grove, CA: Brooks/Cole.

Franklin, C. and Jordan, C. (1999). *Family practice: Brief systems methods for social work*. Pacific Grove, CA: Brooks/Cole.

Hamilton, G. (1950). *Theory and practice of social casework,* Second edition. New York: Columbia University Press.

Janzen, C. and Harris, O. (1997). *Family treatment in social work practice,* Third edition. Itasca, IL: F. E. Peacock.

Kilpatrick, A. and Holland, T. (1999). *Working with families: An integrative model by level of need,* Second edition. Needham Heights, MA: Allyn & Bacon.

Mayer, R. (1985). *Policy and program planning: A developmental perspective.* Englewood Cliffs, NJ: Prentice Hall.

Netting, F. E., Kettner, P. M., and McMurtry, S. L. (1993). *Social work macro practice.* New York: Longman.

Parad, H. (Ed.) (1965). *Crisis intervention: Selected readings.* New York: Family Service Association of America.

Pardeck, J. T. and Yuen, F. K. O. (1997). A family health approach to social work practice. *Family Therapy, 24*(2), 115-128.

Pardeck, J. T. and Yuen, F. K. O. (Eds.) (1999). *Family health: A holistic approach to social work practice.* Westport, CT: Auburn House.

Pardeck, J. T., Yuen, F. K. O., Daley, J., and Hawkins, C. (1998). Social work assessment and intervention through family health practice. *Family Therapy, 25*(1), 25-39.

Payne, M. (1997). *Modern social work theory,* Second edition. Chicago: Lyceum.

Perlman, H. H. (1957). *Social casework: A problem-solving process.* Chicago: University of Chicago Press.

Reid, W. (2002). Knowledge for direct social work practice: An analysis of trends. *Social Service Review, (76)*1, 6-33.

Reid, W. and Epstein, L. (1972). *Task-centered casework.* New York: Columbia University Press.

Richmond, M. (1917). *Social diagnosis.* New York: Free Press.

Rooney, R. H. (1992). *Strategies for work with involuntary clients.* New York: Columbia University Press.

Rothman, J. and Sager, J. S. (1998). *Case management: Integrating individual and community practice,* Second edition. Needham Heights, MA: Allyn & Bacon.

Snyder, W. (1992). Seeing the troubled adolescent in context: Family systems theory and practice. In W. Snyder and T. Ooms (Eds.), *Empowering families, helping adolescents: Family-centered treatment of adolescents with alcohol, drug abuse, and mental health problems* (pp. 13-37). Washington, DC: U.S. Government Printing Office, Office for Treatment Improvement, Department of Health and Human Services.

Walsh, J. (2000). *Clinical case management with persons having mental illness: A relationship-based perspective.* Pacific Grove, CA: Brooks/Cole.

Woods, M. and Hollis, F. (1990). *Casework: A psychosocial therapy,* Fourth edition. New York: McGraw-Hill.

Yuen, F. K. O. (2003). Critical concerns for family health practice. In F. K. O. Yuen, G. J. Skibinski, and J. T. Pardeck (Eds.), *Family health social work practice:*

A knowledge and skills casebook (pp. 19-40). Binghamton, NY: The Haworth Press.

Yuen, F. K. O. and Pardeck, J. T. (1999). A family health approach to social work practice. In J. T. Pardeck and F. K. O. Yuen (Eds.), *Family health: A holistic approach to social work practice* (pp. 1-16). Westport, CT: Auburn House.

Yuen, F. K. O. and Skibinski, G. J. (2003). Family health social work practice: Summary. In F. K. O. Yuen, G. J. Skibinski, and J. T. Pardeck (Eds.), *Family health social work practice: A knowledge and skills casebook* (pp. 203-212). Binghamton, NY: The Haworth Press.

Yuen, F. K. O. and Terao, K. (2003). *Practical grant writing and program evaluation.* Pacific Grove, CA: Brooks/Cole.

SECTION I:
PRACTICE INTERVENTIONS

Chapter 2

Forensic Social Work and Child Sexual Abuse: Family Health Practice and Institutional Constraints

Gregory J. Skibinski
George E. Connor

INTRODUCTION

Forensic social work, defined here as the professional use of the court and legal system to facilitate social work practice, is a seldom researched but often discussed area of social work practice. In this chapter, three models of legal/treatment intervention strategies of child sexual abuse are presented. These models are consistent with the family health perspective and are discussed in terms of developmental influences.

Child sexual abuse cases are reported at an alarming rate and are considered one of the most repugnant crimes. The majority of states have made most forms of child sexual abuse a felony (Bulkley, 1982). Conventional wisdom suggests that felony prosecution is suitable. Many professionals know, however, that it is often detrimental for a number of reasons. First, it is easier to have a case dismissed than to achieve a conviction. As Box 2.1 illustrates, seven steps are required to obtain a conviction, but a dismissal can come at almost any phase of the process.

Legal professionals know that felony convictions are hard to achieve because validation is difficult. For example, physical evidence is rare and testimony to the facts is usually limited to the partic-

BOX 2.1. Common steps in the traditional felony hearing procedure.

1. Offense reported to law enforcement/investigation
   Unfounded/no suspect ——————————> Out of system
   Founded (Arrest warrant issued)
2. Arrest and booking
   Processed pending court appearance
3. Initial court appearance (Probable charges)
   Charges dismissed——————————————> Out of system
   Probable cause
       Guilty ————————————————————> Sentenced
       No contest ——————————————————> Sentenced
       Not guilty
4. Preliminary hearing (May be waived)
   No probable cause ——————————————> Out of system
   Probable cause (Formal charges)
       Guilty ————————————————————> Sentenced
       No contest ——————————————————> Sentenced
       Not guilty
5. Grand jury (May precede or supersede preliminary hearing)
   No probable cause ——————————————> Out of system
   Probable cause (Formal charges)
       Guilty ————————————————————> Sentenced
       No contest ——————————————————> Sentenced
       Not guilty
6. Arraignment (Defendant's response to formal charges)
       Guilty ————————————————————> Sentenced
       No contest ——————————————————> Sentenced
       Not guilty ——————————————————> Set for trial
7. Trial
       Not guilty verdict ——————————————> Out of system
       Guilty verdict ————————————————> Sentenced

ipants. Finally, various political and professional constraints inhibit the creation and implementation of effective intervention strategies. Family health social workers know how difficult it is to keep offenders in treatment unless legal leverage is used. Although a felony conviction may "solve" the criminal case, other family crises may emerge for this already dysfunctional family. Throughout many years of discussion, and trial and error, alternatives to traditional felony prosecutions for first-time offenders in cases of child sexual abuse have developed.

The programs described in this chapter were implemented in three counties in Wisconsin (Eau Claire, Dane, and Milwaukee). They represent the range of child sexual abuse felony diversion strategies used in the state. The first, the Late Diversion Program, utilizes a near-traditional litigation style of diverting the accused only after the arraignment. The Early Diversion Program provides for a prelegal exit of the accused from the system early in the process. Finally, the Mid-Term Diversion Program is a compromise between the other two programs. The Early and Mid-Term Diversion Programs also held simultaneous juvenile court hearings to protect the interests of the victim and families. The text describes the three programs, which Table 2.1 summarizes.

TABLE 2.1. Summary of innovative program characteristics.

Characteristic	Diversion Programs		
	Late	Mid-Term	Early
Offender arrested	Yes	No	No
Charged	Yes	Yes	No
Hearing	Through arraignment	Through initial	None
Plea	Guilty at arraignment	Guilty at initial	N/A
Record after successful treatment	Felony	Arrest	None
Juvenile petition	No	Yes	Yes
Jail	Yes	No	No
Probation	Until victim is 18 years old	No	No
Treatment delivery	After arraignment hearing	After initial hearing	Before legal action
Offender treatment	Required	Required	Required
Victim and family treatment	No provisions	Routine	Routine
Identified client(s)	Offender	Offender, victim, family	Offender, victim, family

TYPES OF DIVERSION PROGRAMS

Late Diversion Program

In this small (population 79,000) industrial community (in Eau Claire County), child sexual abuse professionals determined that their intervention strategies lacked coordination. Social workers and the district attorney developed a package of services consistent with the available resources.

The county held a traditional felony trial to provide treatment and minimal punishment if the assailant pled guilty at the arraignment. Procedurally, the authorities arrested and charged the alleged perpetrator. The accused entered a plea of guilty at the arraignment since the social worker and district attorney believed the accused was not dangerous *and* was treatable. If the judge accepted the plea, the offender would receive (1) up to nine months of jail time, (2) probation until the victim's eighteenth birthday, and (3) treatment. The only other accepted plea would be not guilty. If subsequently convicted, the offender would be sentenced to prison.

A juvenile court petition was not routinely filed, as the victims and their families were not part of the planned intervention package. Social work services and counseling were available at the request of the victims and their families.

Mid-Term Diversion Program

In this moderately sized (population 324,000) university and state capital city (in Dane County), the alleged offender was requested to appear at a pretrial conference. Failure to appear would result in an arrest and a traditional felony hearing. The purpose of the pretrial conference was to determine the offender's potential for treatment. If thought to be treatable, the accused would be charged as a child molester, then he or she would plead guilty at the initial appearance and would thus be diverted from further prosecution into a preexisting treatment program. The plea would be vacated upon the successful completion of the treatment program. If sufficient progress was not made, a guilty plea would be entered again, and the convict would be sentenced as a felon.

The victim and other family members were expected to receive treatment and other services provided by a juvenile court petition that would be routinely filed.

Early Diversion Program

As in the Mid-Term Diversion Program, the accused in this large (population 965,000), urban, industrialized county (Milwaukee) was not arrested but invited to a pretrial conference. Again, failure to appear would result in an arrest and a traditional felony hearing. If the district attorney, the social worker, and the arresting officer determined the alleged offender to be treatable, he or she would be diverted into a treatment program *without* being charged. Successful completion of the treatment program would end the case. No record would be kept except to enter the accused offender's name into a file as a successfully treated, first-time offender. Treatment failure would initiate a traditional felony hearing.

As in the Mid-Term Diversion Program, a petition would be routinely filed in juvenile court, providing victim and family services as necessary.

The purpose of this chapter is to examine the various constraints on a family health social worker in developing legal and treatment intervention strategies for cases of child sexual abuse. The constraints are legal, political, and professional. Of the three, the professional constraints may be the most important to focus on because they operate in a world defined by the other two.

LEGAL CONSTRAINTS

Three sets of legal constraints inhibit the development of child sexual abuse intervention programs for family health social workers: lack of physical evidence, witness trauma, and precedents.

Most forms of child sexual abuse are felonies; a few are misdemeanors. All are crimes. As such, offender conviction would seem beneficial and simple. However, due to a lack of physical evidence in most cases and the inherent problems with eyewitness testimony to secretive acts, convictions in a traditional court of law are difficult to obtain.

For violent crimes such as rape society attempts to protect both the victim from revictimization and the general population from future assaults. Protective mechanisms include arrests, restraining orders, and imprisonment (Robin, 1984).

In child sexual assault cases, there also exists the concern of decreasing the secondary victimization to children that may result from those protection attempts, for example, multiple interviews and testifying in court (Berliner and Barbieri, 1984; Costin, Bell, and Downs, 1991; Cross, Whitcomb, and De Vos, 1995; Dziech and Schudson, 1991; Eatman and Bulkley, 1986; Fargason et al., 1994; Gothard, 1987; King, Hunter, and Runyon, 1988; Koszuth, 1991; *Maryland v. Craig,* 1990; Saywitz and Nathanson, 1993). Prosecution requires proof beyond a reasonable doubt based on physical evidence and the child's testimony. Both require the child's cooperation (e.g., medical examinations; interviews with police, social workers, and the district attorney; and court testimony). Although this process parallels the ordeal of adult rape victims, it may be even more psychologically harmful for children.

Physical Evidence

Research indicates that it is very difficult to confirm child sexual abuse via medical diagnosis. For example, in a study of alleged penile or digital penetration by Muram (1989) the "examiner described normal appearing genitalia . . . or non-specific abnormalities" in 39 percent of his cases (p. 211). Paradise (1989) found false positives in vaginal diameter tests for two-thirds (penile penetration) to three-fourths (digital penetration) of reported child sexual assaults. Similarly, the transmission of anogenital warts is not diagnostic of child sexual assault (Hanson et al., 1989).

Not only is medical assessment an uncertain diagnostic tool (Skibinski and Nelson-Gardell, 2000) but the presence of physical evidence is unlikely in child sexual abuse cases. This finding should not be surprising, as child sexual assault is usually a coercive rather than violent offense and orifice penetration typically occurs only after a long history of abuse.

Hanson et al. (1989) concluded that the diagnosis of child sexual abuse must be "made on history rather than examination" (p. 225). Other research (Cupoli and Sewell, 1988) supports this conclusion. Many nonphysical indicators also exist. Box 2.2 lists five sets of indicators. Although a multidisciplinary assessment is clearly indicated

BOX 2.2. Nonphysical indicators of child sexual abuse.

Medical

1. Pregnancy
2. Sexually transmitted diseases
3. Tears or bleeding in the groin area
4. Enlargements or swelling in the vaginal area
5. Bruises
6. Spermatozoa
7. Broken hymen
8. Difficulty in sitting or walking

Behavioral

9. Sexual content in child's play or other activities
10. Seductive behavior
11. Promiscuous behavior
12. Regressive behavior
13. Withdrawal
14. Excessive clinging
15. Mother-daughter role reversal
16. Pseudomaturity
17. Excessive or compulsive masturbation
18. Running away from home
19. Social difficulties

Cognitive and affective

20. Precocious knowledge
21. Sexual knowledge learned from experience
22. Affective response consistent with the trauma
23. Depression
24. Powerlessness
25. Anger
26. Embarrassment
27. Shame
28. Fear of a particular person or situation
29. Fear and anxiety about the opposite sex
30. Fear and confusion about sex

(continued)

(continued)

Psychophysiological

31. Sleeping disorders
32. Eating disorders

Other

33. Elements of secrecy
34. Elements of pressure or coercion
35. Hesitancy to discuss the abuse allegations
36. Opportunity factors

Sources: Compiled and adapted from Finkelhor et al., 1990; Bays and Chadwick, 1993; Sgroi, 1982; Faller, 1988; Brassard et al., 1983; Jiles, 1980; Conte and Berliner, 1981.

(Brant and Tisza, 1977; Herbert, 1987; Shamroy, 1980; Sink, 1986; Terrell, 1977), many cases hinge on the child's testimony.

Testimony

Child sexual abuse is an assault, but rarely are there witnesses (Costin, Bell, and Downs, 1991). Available testimony about this private, secretive assault is often limited to the victim and the offender. The offender is not likely to testify against himself or herself (especially in the absence of evidence), and the victim is often afraid to retell the story. The process may be even more painful if the accused is a family member (Costin, Bell, and Downs, 1991). Given the nature of child sexual abuse, a witness will be more credible if the testimony uncovers

1. multiple incidents over time;
2. progression of the sexual activity;
3. elements of secrecy;
4. elements of pressure or coercion;
5. explicit details and precocious knowledge; and
6. a consistent, logical story (appropriate to child's age) (compiled and adapted from Berliner and Conte, 1993; Faller, 1988; Sgroi, 1982).

Although the text of the Sixth Amendment to the U.S. Constitution states clearly that "In all criminal prosecutions, the accused shall enjoy the right to . . . be confronted with the witnesses against him," the application of this constitutional provision is problematic in cases involving abuse victims classified as minors. For example, the testimony of children is a potential problem since the competence and credibility of the child may be questioned (Dziech and Schudson, 1991; Faller, 1988; Myers, 1993; Ordway, 1983; Sagatun and Edwards, 1995; Saywitz and Nathanson, 1993), and most assailants are either biological parents or parental figures (e.g., stepparent, foster parent, parent's girfriend or boyfriend) (Skibinski, 1990), making testifying difficult (Costin, Bell, and Downs, 1991). The process may be further complicated if the child is traumatically bonded to (i.e., ironically protective of) the offender (deYoung and Lowry, 1992). Thus, the offender's arrest, detention, and imprisonment may protect the child and society, but the trauma to the child and family may outweigh the benefits.

The case of *Coy v. Iowa* (1988) offers a cogent yet poignant illustration. Two thirteen-year-old girls were sexually abused in a makeshift tent in one of their backyards. Because there was "only circumstantial evidence against" the accused (Coy), the girls' "testimony became crucial" (Alderman and Kennedy, 1991, p. 230). As reported by the county prosecutor, Gary Rolfes, the girls were "horrified at the idea" of testifying at the trial and "wouldn't come near the courthouse" (Alderman and Kennedy, 1991, p. 231). After being denied the opportunity to testify via closed-circuit television, the girls testified in open court behind a screen that permitted the accused to see them without the girls being able to see the accused. As will be discussed, this arrangement led to the overturning of Coy's conviction by the U.S. Supreme Court. Four years later, as Iowa proceeded with a retrial, the girls refused to participate. When the new county prosecutor, Bruce Ingham, dropped the case, he explained: "Our attitude is pretty much victim oriented here in that if the victim doesn't want to go forward, neither do we" (Alderman and Kennedy, 1991, p. 240).

Aside from providing insight into the further victimization of the victims, the *Coy* case also illustrates the importance of physical evidence in sexual abuse cases. Because "parts of the girls' description seemed to indicate that Coy was not the assailant," solid physical evidence would have enhanced the prosecution's case (Alderman and

Kennedy, 1991, p. 230). However, the physical evidence (finger-prints, hair samples, urine samples, flashlight batteries) could not be positively linked to the accused. The absence of physical evidence necessitated the testimony of the girls, regardless of the trauma it might engender (Alderman and Kennedy, 1991).

Although utilizing children as witnesses in sexual abuse cases is within the range of police powers reserved by the Tenth Amendment for the states, the federal courts have established some precedents with respect to this issue. Further complicated by the trauma inflicted on a minor witness, the arguments that arise in these cases lay at the nexus of two distinct legal issues: hearsay and confrontation. Out-of-court statements are usually not admissible as hearsay evidence. However, the U.S. Supreme Court has indicated that when evidence is "only available in the form of hearsay . . . the rules of evidence may allow admissions of such out-of-court statements" (Alderman and Kennedy, 1991, p. 397). "May allow" is the crucial variable, because the Court has never clearly spelled out the grounds for exception (Alderman and Kennedy, 1991). The U.S. Supreme Court has said that "if a procedure is found to be 'inherently prejudicial,' a guilty verdict will not be upheld if the procedure was not necessary to further an essential state interest" (Alderman and Kennedy, 1991, p. 232). The Court has, in effect, forced prosecutors to choose between the rights of the accused and the rights of the victim. This dichotomy can be illustrated by the Court's opinions in *Coy* and the subsequent case, *Maryland v. Craig* (1990).

Writing for the majority in *Coy*, Justice Antonin Scalia cited former Justice John Marshall Harlan while asserting that "simply as a matter of English [the confrontation clause] confers at least 'a right to meet face to face all those who appear and give evidence at trial'" (Alderman and Kennedy, 1991, p. 238). Addressing the specific issue of trauma, the Court concluded that "face-to-face presence may, unfortunately, upset the truthful rape victim or abused child; but by the same token it may confound and undo the false accuser, or reveal the child coached by a malevolent adult." Rather than finding fault with the trial judge, the majority fixed blame squarely on the shoulders of the Iowa state legislature who "had created a 'legislatively imposed presumption of trauma' of *all* child witnesses" instead of stipulating that an "individualized finding that these particular witnesses under these circumstances need this kind of special protection" was warranted (Alderman and Kennedy, 1991, p. 239). Although the *Coy* ruling settled the case, it did not resolve the underlying dilemma.

Dissenting from the *Coy* majority were Justice Harry A. Blackmun and Chief Justice William H. Rehnquist. Recognizing that "the prosecution of child sex-abuses poses substantial difficulties because of the emotional trauma frequently suffered by child witnesses who must testify about the sexual assaults they have suffered" (*Coy v. Iowa,* 108 Sup. Ct. 2798 p. 2808) they maintained that

> the fear and trauma associated with a child's testimony in front of the defendant have two serious identifiable consequences: They may cause psychological injury to the child, and they may so overwhelm the child as to prevent the possibility of effective testimony, thereby undermining the truth-finding function of the trial itself. (*Coy v. Iowa,* 108 Sup. Ct. 2798 p. 2809)

Moreover, the two justices maintained that it was entirely appropriate for the Iowa legislature to make exceptions to the confrontation clause.

Striking more of a middle ground, Justice Sandra Day O'Connor wrote a separate, concurring opinion. She noted her agreement with the majority in that "the Confrontation Clause was violated in this case." However, Justice O'Connor acknowledged that "child abuse is a problem of disturbing proportions" and recognized the states that had "determined that a child victim may suffer trauma from exposure to the harsh atmosphere of the typical courtroom." In acknowledging the relationship between sexual abuse and testimony she offered hope for future exceptions to the confrontation clause: "I wish to make clear that nothing in today's decision necessarily dooms efforts by state legislatures to protect child witnesses" (*Coy v. Iowa,* 108 Sup. Ct. 2798 p. 2804). Although Justice Scalia disagreed with this interpretation, it did offer prophetic insight into the outcome of the next significant case dealing with sexual abuse and child witnesses.

The 1990 decision in *Maryland v. Craig* began by recognizing the legitimate state interest in safeguarding child witnesses in sexual abuse cases. The Court held that although the confrontation clause was "made applicable to the States through the Fourteenth Amendment" (*Maryland v. Craig* 110 Sup. Ct. 3157 p. 3162), the clause does not "guarantee criminal defendants the absolute right to a face-to-face meeting with witnesses against them at trial" (*Maryland v. Craig*

110 Sup. Ct. 3157 p. 3163). Writing for the Court majority, Justice O'Connor concluded that

> where necessary to protect a child witness from trauma that would be caused by testifying in the physical presences of the defendant, at least where such trauma would impair the child's ability to communicate, the Confrontation Clause does not prohibit use of a procedure that, despite absence of face-to-face confrontation, ensures the reliability of the evidence by subjecting it to rigorous adversarial testing and thereby preserves the essence of effective confrontation. (*Maryland v. Craig* 110 Sup. Ct. 3157 p. 3171)

The shift in the Court majority, a brief two years after the *Coy* decision, can be explained by three points contained in the majority opinion. From a legal standpoint, the Court insisted that, unlike the blanket trauma assumed by the Iowa statute in *Coy*, the Maryland statute mandated that "the trial court must hear evidence and determine whether" the special procedure "is necessary to protect the welfare of the particular child witness" (*Maryland v. Craig* 110 Sup. Ct. 3157 p. 3169). With regard to federalism, the Court recognized that "a significant majority of States ha[d] enacted statutes to protect child witnesses from the trauma of giving testimony," attesting "to the widespread belief in the importance of such a policy" (*Maryland v. Craig* 110 Sup. Ct. 3157 p. 3167). Finally, the Court concluded that its decision was "buttressed by a growing body of academic literature documenting the psychological trauma suffered by child abuse victims who must testify in court" (*Maryland v. Craig* 110 Sup. Ct. 3157 p. 3168).

Categorically rejecting the majority's opinion, Justice Scalia offered a fairly scathing dissent. Joined by Justices William J. Brennan, Thurgood Marshall, and John Paul Stevens, Scalia argued that "seldom has this Court failed so conspicuously to sustain a categorical guarantee of the Constitution against the tide of prevailing current opinion" (*Maryland v. Craig* 110 Sup. Ct. 3157 p. 3171). The dissenters' position is clear. The majority maintains that the state interest "in the physical and psychological well-being of child abuse victims . . . outweighs the explicit text of the Constitution." Scalia's opinion simply counters: "That is not so" (*Maryland v. Craig* 110 Sup Ct. 3157 p. 3175).

Although the shifting Court majority offers guidance to states and their subsidiary jurisdictions, one cannot escape the certain degree of irony inherent in the majority opinion in *Maryland v. Craig*. Clearly the opinion lends credence to the family health perspective mode of intervention. Nevertheless, while seeking to protect the victims of child abuse, the establishment of another layer of judicial procedures subjects victims of child abuse to additional legal, and potentially traumatic, scrutiny.

POLITICAL CONSTRAINTS

Family health intervention by social workers in child sexual abuse cases is further impacted by the political constraints of the local political system. According to Elazar (1970), the local political system can be defined as

> the organized sum of the political institutions which function in a given locality to provide it with the bundle of governmental services and activities that can be manipulated locally to serve the local needs in light of local values. Hence a locality becomes a community insofar as its existence is defined by its organization for political—or civil—purposes. (p. 5)

Although this definition applies equally to Milwaukee, Dane, and Eau Claire counties, Elazar (1970) reminds us that it is "necessary to determine the character and limits of each specific civil community, based on certain common politically significant components shared by them all." These components are as follows:

1. formally established local governments (municipality, school districts, and so on);
2. local agencies of the state and federal governments;
3. nongovernmental public bodies (chambers of commerce, PTAs);
4. political parties that mobilize and structure political activity;
5. system of interest groups that function in the local political arena;
6. shared public concerns as reflected in the bundle of public services and activities provided locally; and
7. written constitutional material and unwritten political tradition. (p. 6)

The individuality of each civil community is determined by the unique combination of these components. More important, each community's unique combination leads to variability in public policies. This is especially true with respect to policies and procedures dealing with child sexual abuse. Regarding the treatment of sex abuse offenders, the most important of these components are the formally established governments, the local agencies of the state government, and the shared public concerns of the community.

In regard to local governments and the role of state agencies, issues of jurisdiction are paramount. Elazar (1970) has observed that "the urban civil community almost invariably has a city at its core, no matter how much its population and political system may transcend the formal municipal limits" (p. 6). This observation holds true for the three counties under consideration in this chapter. Although the city of Milwaukee dominates Milwaukee County, it is not the sole political entity. Milwaukee County also includes eighteen other municipalities. Similarly, Dane County encompasses fifty-nine towns, villages, and cities along with the more populous state capitol, Madison. Unlike her sister counties, Eau Claire consists of only the county seat, Eau Claire, and ten other towns. Nevertheless, similar to Milwaukee and Madison, the city of Eau Claire clearly overshadows political affairs in the county. One additional reality of political geography for Eau Claire is also worth noting. Although the city may lie at the heart of an urban civil community, it is important to remember that "county lines almost invariably mark its potential outer limits" (Elazar, 1970, p. 6).

Although local agencies of state government are present in all three counties, this presence is not uniform. Without question and for obvious reasons, the state is the most visible in Dane County. As one would expect, the state's presence is more muted in Eau Claire County. After Dane County, Milwaukee County has the most significant number of state offices and, therefore, a very visible state presence. The Wisconsin Department of Administration's Division of Administrative Services oversees the State Prosecutor's Office. As indicated by the department's title, the state provides administrative assistance to district attorneys across the state. It is imperative, given the local variations in political culture, to note that the seventy-one district attorneys in Wisconsin are popularly elected at the county level.

The set of shared public concerns varies naturally from community to community. However, within regions and states, it can be said that a dominant political culture exists. Of the three political cultures identified by Elazar (1970), only the moralistic and individualistic apply to Wisconsin. In an individualistic political culture, "the political order is conceived as a marketplace in which the primary public relationships are products of bargaining among individuals and groups acting out of self-interest" (p. 258). Elazar (1970) notes further that the individualistic political culture "places a premium on limiting community intervention" and "public officials in the individualistic political culture are not normally willing to initiate new programs or open up new areas of government activity on their own initiative" (p. 260). "They will do so when they perceive an overwhelming public demand for them to act, but only then" (Elazar, 1970, p. 261).

According to Elazar (1970), in a moralistic political culture,

> the political order is conceived to be a commonwealth—a state in which the whole people have an undivided interest—in which the citizens cooperated in an effort to create and maintain the best government in order to implement certain shared principles. (pp. 258-259)

In this type of culture, "individualism is tempered by a general commitment to utilizing communal power to intervene into the sphere of 'private' activities when it is necessary to do so for the public good or the well-being of the community" (Elazar, 1970, p. 262). Contrary to the individualistic political culture, "the moralistic political culture creates a greater commitment to active government interventions into the economic and social life of the community" (Elazar, 1970, p. 263). According to these defining characteristics, Elazar identified Wisconsin as a state with a moralistic political culture: "The sense of communal responsibility that was part of the mainstream culture of Wisconsin's dominant migratory currents has become rooted in the political culture of the state and in most of its civil communities" (p. 357). As compared to other states, including those in the upper Midwest, the data suggest that "state government in Wisconsin has acted more frequently and with greater effect" and that Wisconsin has "gone further toward centralizing regulatory and social services than all but a handful in the nation" (Elazar, 1970, p. 359). Elazar qualifies this conclusion by stating that Wisconsin is not free of intrastate conflict and admitting that state and local conflicts do exist. However, these conflicts arise because of the implementation of specific programs, not because of policy.

One might imagine that a family health approach to instances of child sexual abuse would be a natural fit in a state or civil community with a moralistic political culture. However, as the three-county data indicate, this is not the case. Defined by a "sense of communal responsibility" (Elazar, 1970, p. 357), the moralistic political culture can be interpreted by prosecutors in terms of punishing child sexual offenders to protect the greater community from further and future harm. This same "communal responsibility" can also be translated into the recognition of the child victim as part of the civil community. This recognition is consistent with Bruce Ingham's refusal to retry the *Coy* case. Serving the best interests of the child victim can be equated with serving the long-term interests of the community. Similarly, one might assume that criminal justice policy in an individual political culture might be more focused on punishment. Again, however, the data are mixed. Eau Claire, Dane, and Milwaukee counties exhibit some individualistic components. In this way, Milwaukee's political culture is related to other large urban cities in the Midwest. Nevertheless, the Milwaukee County data indicate that prosecutors utilize a somewhat communal approach to the prosecution of child sexual abuse offenders. Elazar's (1970) theory explains these data by noting that "even those groups which fall within the range of the individualistic political culture share a strong commitment to (or at least acceptance of) activist government" (p. 358).

PROFESSIONAL CONSTRAINTS

In response to these obstacles and constraints, professionals have developed the three family health intervention systems described previously. The systems differ on a variety of issues, but most important, they focus on controlling the offenders and treating those in need.

Controlling the Offender

Criminal prosecutions attempt to control the offender and protect the community through imprisonment. However, prosecution is a long process (Martone, Jaudes, and Cavins, 1996), and long-term imprisonment is unlikely (MacFarlane and Bulkley, 1982). Due to the attractiveness of plea bargains alternative intervention programs may provide faster and more certain control of offenders than criminal prosecution (Cross, Whitcomb, and De Vos, 1995; Martone, Jaudes, and Cavins, 1996; Oberlander, 1995). Diversion strategies attempt to protect the child and control the offender with a minimum of legal red tape. Offenders may find diversion programs attractive since they may avoid criminal prosecutions as well as publicity. Society might find them more attractive as the alleged offenders (and therefore the community) may benefit from treatment.

Treating Those in Need

Intrafamilial child sexual abuse is indicative of family dysfunction (Fleming, Mullen, and Bammer, 1997; Frude, 1982; Giaretto, 1982; Leifer, Shapiro, and Kassem, 1993; Peterson, Basta, and Dykstra, 1993; Salter, 1988). The sexual abuse only exacerbates the problems. Nonabusing mothers are also affected (Newberger et al., 1993) and struggle to respond appropriately to the incident (Humphreys, 1992). Family treatment is often proposed, but present service delivery systems are often insensitive to the needs of mothers and their children (Carter, 1993). In criminal prosecutions, treatment of the offender is unlikely to occur because the purpose of the hearing is to mete out justice, not rectify personal or family ills. Furthermore, the accused is the only party to the legal action, making court-ordered treatment for the victim and his or her family atypical as well.

Legal/treatment intervention programs modeled after MacFarlane and Bulkley's (1982) work use rehabilitation and the threat of incarceration as the primary mechanisms of intervention, requiring mandatory treatment for alleged offenders with counseling and other services offered to the victim and the victim's family. The purpose is to minimize family dysfunction, rectify offender problems, and support and protect the child.

CONCLUSION

Child sexual abuse intervention programs that integrate treatment and legal procedures can take a multitude of forms. Briefly described in this chapter were three different child sexual abuse diversionary models that represent the range of legal/treatment strategies developed primarily for use with first-time intrafamilial offenders.

Although the goals of adversarial and diversionary intervention are similar, the strategies and techniques to achieve these goals differ markedly. These and other imaginative legal/treatment strategies for intrafamilial child sexual abuse cases have been developed in communities nationwide by district attorneys, social workers, and other child abuse professionals (Bander, Fein, and Bishop, 1982; Bulkley, 1981; Conte and Berliner, 1981; Cramer, 1985; Fein and Bishop, 1987; Giaretto, 1982; Whitcomb, 1985; Young, 1988).

The major goals of child sexual abuse litigation strategies are to (1) *control* the offender, (2) *protect* the victim from the offender and further victimization (i.e., testimony), and (3) *treat* the victim(s) (and rehabilitate the offender). It appears that social workers, in cooperation with other professionals, accomplish these goals in various ways and these approaches have many advantages. Justice may be quicker, the child and family can receive treatment, the offender can be controlled, and the child can be protected from revictimization and secondary victimization. Most family health social workers in child sexual abuse cases base their intervention strategies on sound professional judgment.

REFERENCES

Alderman, E. and Kennedy, C. (1991). *In our defense: The Bill of Rights in action.* New York: Avon Books.

Bander, K., Fein, E., and Bishop, G. (1982). Child sex abuse treatment: Some barriers to program operation. *Child Abuse and Neglect: The International Journal,* 6, 185-191.

Bays, J. and Chadwick, D. (1993). Medical diagnosis of the sexually abused child. *Child Abuse and Neglect: The International Journal, 17,* 91-110.

Berliner, L. and Barbieri, M. K. (1984). The testimony of the child victim of sexual assault. *Journal of Social Issues, 40*(2), 125-137.

Berliner, L. and Conte, J. R. (1993). Sexual abuse evaluations: Conceptual and empirical obstacles. *Child Abuse and Neglect: The International Journal, 17*(1), 111-125.

Brant, R. S. T. and Tisza, V. B. (1977). The sexually misused child. *American Journal of Orthopsychiatry, 47*(1), 80-90.

Brassard, M. R., Tyler, A., and Kehle, T. J. (1983). Sexually abused children: Identification and suggestions for intervention. *School Psychology Review, 12*(1), 93-97.

Bulkley, J. (Ed.) (1981). *Innovations in the prosecution of child sexual abuse cases.* Washington, DC: American Bar Association.

Bulkley, J. (1982). *Recommendations for improving legal intervention in intrafamily child sexual abuse cases.* Washington, DC: American Bar Association.

Carter, B. (1993). Child sexual abuse: Impact on mothers. *AFFILIA: Journal of Women and Social Work, 8*(1), 72-90.

Conte, J. R. and Berliner, L. (1981). Prosecution of the offender in cases of sexual assault against children. *Victimology: An International Journal, 6*(1-4), 102-109.

Costin, L. B., Bell, C. J., and Downs, S. W. (1991). *Child welfare: Policies and practice,* Fourth edition. White Plains, NY: Longman.

Coy v. Iowa, 108 Sup. Ct. 2798 (1988).

Cramer, R. E., Jr. (1985). The district attorney as a mobilizer in a community approach to child sexual abuse. *University of Miami Law Review, 40*(1), 209-216.

Cross, T. P., Whitcomb, D., and De Vos, E. (1995). Criminal justice outcomes of prosecution of child sexual abuse. *Child Abuse and Neglect: The International Journal, 19*(12), 1431-1442.

Cupoli, J. M. and Sewell, P. M. (1988). One thousand fifty-nine children with a chief complaint of sexual abuse. *Child Abuse and Neglect: The International Journal, 12,* 151-162.

deYoung, M. and Lowry, J. A. (1992). Traumatic bonding: Clinical implications in incest. *Child Welfare, 71*(2), 165-175.

Dziech, B. W. and Schudson, C. B. (1991). *On trial: America's courts and their treatment of sexually abused children,* Second edition. Boston: Beacon Press.

Eatman, R. and Bulkley, J. (Eds.) (1986). *Protecting child victim/witnesses: Sample laws and materials.* Washington, DC: American Bar Association.

Elazar, D. J. (1970). *Cities of the prairie.* New York: Basic Books.

Faller, K. C. (1988). Criteria for judging the credibility of children's statements about their sexual abuse. *Child Welfare, 67,* 389-401.

Fargason, C. A., Jr., Barnes, D., Schneider, D., and Galloway, B. W. (1994). Enhancing multi-agency collaboration in the management of child sexual abuse. *Child Abuse and Neglect: The International Journal, 18*(10), 859-869.

Fein, E. and Bishop, G. V. (1987). Child sexual abuse: Treatment for the offender. *Social Casework, 68*(2), 122-124.

Finkelhor, D., Hotaling, G., Lewis, I. A., and Smith, C. (1990). Sexual abuse in a national survey of adult men and women: Prevalence, characteristics, and risk factors. *Child Abuse and Neglect, 14*(1), 19-28.

Fleming, J., Mullen, P., and Bammer, G. (1997). A study of potential risk factors for sexual abuse in childhood. *Child Abuse and Neglect: The International Journal, 21*(1), 49-58.

Frude, N. (1982). The sexual nature of sexual abuse: A review of the literature. *Child Abuse and Neglect: The International Journal, 6,* 211-223.

Giaretto, H. (1982). A comprehensive child sexual abuse treatment program. *Child Abuse and Neglect: The International Journal, 6,* 263-278.

Gothard, S. (1987). The admissibility of evidence in child sexual abuse cases. *Child Welfare, 66*(1), 13-24.

Hanson, R. M., Glasson, M., McCrossin, I., and Rogers, M. (1989). Anogenital warts in childhood. *Child Abuse and Neglect: The International Journal, 13,* 225-233.

Herbert, C. P. (1987). Expert medical assessment in determining probability of alleged child sexual abuse. *Child Abuse and Neglect: The International Journal, 11,* 213-221.

Humphreys, C. (1992). Disclosure of child sexual assault: Implications for mothers. *Australian Social Work, 45*(3), 27-35.

Jiles, D. (1980). Problems in the assessment of sexual abuse referrals. In W. M. Holder (Ed.), *Sexual abuse of children: Implications for treatment* (pp. 59-64). Englewood, CO: The American Humane Association.

King, N. M. P., Hunter, W. M., and Runyon, D. K. (1988). Going to court: The experience of child victims of intrafamilial sexual abuse. *Journal of Health Politics, Policy and Law, 13,* 705-721.

Koszuth, A. M. (1991). Sexually abused child syndrome: Res ipsa loquitur and shifting the burden of proof. *Law and Psychology Review, 15,* 277-297.

Leifer, M., Shapiro, J. P., and Kassem, L. (1993). The impact of maternal history and behavior upon foster placement and adjustment in sexually abused girls. *Child Abuse and Neglect: The International Journal, 17*(6), 755-766.

MacFarlane, K. and Bulkley, J. (1982). Treating child sexual abuse: An overview of current program models. *Social Work and Child Sexual Abuse, 1,* 69-91.

Martone, M., Jaudes, P. K., and Cavins, M. K. (1996). Criminal prosecution of child sexual abuse cases. *Child Abuse and Neglect: The International Journal, 20*(5), 457-464.

Maryland v. Craig, 110 Sup. Ct. 3157 (1990).

Muram, D. (1989). Child sexual abuse: Relationship between sexual acts and genital findings. *Child Abuse and Neglect: The International Journal, 13,* 211-216.

Myers, J. E. B. (1993). Commentary: A call for forensically relevant research. *Child Abuse and Neglect: The International Journal, 17*(5), 613-622.

Newberger, C. M., Gremy, I. M., Waternaux, C. M., and Newberger, E. H. (1993). Mothers of sexually abused children: Trauma and repair in longitudinal perspective. *American Journal of Orthopsychiatry, 63*(1), 92-102.

Oberlander, L. B. (1995). Psycholegal issues in child sexual abuse evaluations: A survey of forensic mental health professionals. *Child Abuse and Neglect: The International Journal, 19*(4), 475-490.

Ordway, D. P. (1983). Reforming judicial procedures for handling parent-child incest. *Child Welfare, 62*(1), 68-75.

Paradise, J. E. (1989). Predictive accuracy and the diagnosis of sexual abuse: A big issue about a little tissue. *Child Abuse and Neglect: The International Journal, 13*, 169-176.

Peterson, R. F., Basta, S. M., and Dykstra, T. A. (1993). Mothers of molested children: Some comparisons of personality characteristics. *Child Abuse and Neglect: The International Journal, 17*(3), 409-418.

Robin, G. D. (1984). *Introduction to the criminal justice system: Principles, procedures, practice,* Second edition. New York: Harper & Row.

Sagatun, I. J. and Edwards, L. P. (1995). *Child abuse and the legal system.* Chicago: Nelson-Hall.

Salter, A. M. (1988). *Treating child sex offenders and victims: A practical guide.* Newbury Park, CA: Sage.

Saywitz, K. J. and Nathanson, R. (1993). Children's testimony and their perceptions of stress in and out of the courtroom. *Child Abuse and Neglect: The International Journal, 17*(5), 613-622.

Sgroi, S. M. (1982). *A handbook of clinical intervention in child sexual abuse.* Lexington, MA: Lexington Books.

Shamroy, J. A. (1980). A perspective on child sexual abuse. *Social Work* (March), 128-131.

Sink, F. (1986). Child sexual abuse: Comprehensive assessment in the pediatric health care setting. *Child Health Care, 15*(2), 108-113.

Skibinski, G. J. (1990). Factors related to the processing of child sexual abuse cases by social workers in three Wisconsin counties (Doctoral dissertation, University of Wisconsin–Madison, 1989). *Dissertation Abstracts International, 50,* 3061A.

Skibinski, G. J. and Nelson-Gardell, D. (2000). Confirming child sexual abuse: Little help from medical examinations. *The SMSU Journal of Public Affairs, 4,* 22-39.

Terrell, M. E. (1977). Identifying the sexually abused child in a medical setting. *Health and Social Work, 2*(4), 113-130.

Whitcomb, D. (1985). *Prosecution of child sexual abuse: Innovations in practice.* Washington, DC: National Institute of Justice.

Young, W. M. (1988). Vermont sexual abuse/assault protocol. In A. C. Salter (Ed.), *Treating child sex offenders and victims: A practical guide* (pp. 254-261). Newbury Park, CA: Sage.

Chapter 3

Using Bibliotherapy in Family Health Social Work Practice with Children of Divorce

John T. Pardeck

INTRODUCTION

Divorce is one of the most common forms of family breakdown in the United States. Divorce continues to increase each year and affects millions of children. Goldenberg and Goldenberg (2000) report that more than 1 million children under the age of eighteen are living in one-parent homes as a result of divorce.

The divorce process is often stressful for both children and parents. Parents who divorce may feel a sense of failure; children may experience, among other things, conflicting loyalties between their divorcing parents. Yet the research evidence concludes that divorce is better (or at least less harmful) for children than remaining in a family system in which parents are engaged in ongoing conflict (Goldenberg and Goldenberg, 2000). Even though divorce helps end the conflict between parents, children of divorce will still have to make the emotional transition from a two-parent to a one-parent family system. Many of these children, if a parent remarries, will experience another major emotional and social transition into a blended family system (Goldenberg and Goldenberg, 2000).

Divorce involves a two-stage process: the predivorce and the postdivorce stages. Divorce has a tendency to be different from other kinds of family breakdown, such as the death of a parent, because both parents usually continue to have contact with their children after divorce. If family breakdown is a result of the death of a parent, obviously the relationship with that parent ends. Children of divorce will often continue the relationship with the parent who leaves the family, typically the father. This ongoing relationship may be difficult for the child as well as the absent parent (Goldstein, Freud, and Solnit, 1973).

FAMILY HEALTH CONSIDERATIONS

It is important to view the family from a family health perspective in order to effectively assess and treat stressors impacting the family. Divorce is a family event that often creates tremendous stress on the family system. The family health perspective helps the practitioner move from a traditional, narrow psychological perspective for understanding the divorce process to a systems level at which interaction and transaction with the environment is considered. By moving away from purely psychological factors to a systems-ecological orientation, all parties are better able to understand the breakdown of the family system due to divorce (Germain, 1979; Pardeck, 1998).

Minuchin (1974) suggests that problems related to family breakdown due to divorce can be dealt with more effectively if families receive help early; dysfunctional family patterns are more difficult to correct the longer the family waits to receive treatment. The family health perspective is in agreement with Minuchin's position on the importance of families receiving help early when confronted with problems such as divorce. The goal of family health social work practice is to enhance the physical, mental, emotional, social, economic, cultural, and spiritual functioning of the family system, which results in the holistic well-being of the family and its members (Pardeck and Yuen, 1999). Stressors on the family system, such as divorce, may have a negative impact on family health. Bibliotherapy is a therapeutic approach that can be helpful in treating families experiencing divorce, particularly the children of these families.

FAMILY HEALTH AND BIBLIOTHERAPY

Bibliotherapy can be a useful approach for helping children deal with psychological problems and various transitions through the family and individual life cycle that may include divorce. Bibliotherapy most simply defined means helping clients—including children—

deal with emotional and adjustment problems, as well as basic developmental needs, through the use of literature (Pardeck, 1998). Bibliotherapy can help children who are unable to verbalize their thoughts and feelings about confronting problems. Books can also help children find alternative solutions to problems through selected children's literature. By reading literature, troubled children can discover how others similar to themselves have confronted problems and solved them. An in-depth review of the research literature by Pardeck (1998) concludes that bibliotherapy can help promote personal growth and development in children and help them deal with various psychological problems. These are all goals consistent with the family health perspective.

GOALS AND PRINCIPLES GUIDING BIBLIOTHERAPY

The treatment goals for working with children through the bibliotherapeutic process include

- teaching positive thinking;
- encouraging free expression of a presenting problem;
- encouraging solutions to a presenting problem; and
- helping children understand the similarities of their problems to those of others.

Watson (1980) concludes that if these goals can be achieved, positive therapeutic change can occur.

Rubin (1978) suggests that clinicians need to be sensitive to certain principles when using bibliotherapy with children. These include the following:

- Practitioners should only use reading materials they are familiar with.
- There must be sensitivity to the length of the reading materials; the practitioner should avoid complex readings with extraneous details and situations.

- The child's presenting problem should be similar to but not necessarily identical to the problem found in the reading material.
- The child's reading level and interests should be known; this information should guide what reading materials are used. If a child cannot read or has reading deficiencies, reading aloud to the child or using audiovisual materials is an effective approach to bibliotherapeutic intervention. For young children, reading aloud is the suggested approach for using literature in treatment. The child's emotional and chronological age must be considered and reflected in the level of sophistication of the reading materials selected.
- Reading materials that express the same feelings or mood as the child's are excellent choices for bibliotherapeutic intervention. This approach is called the *isoprinciple,* which stems from the technique of music and poetry therapy.
- Audiovisual materials should be considered in the bibliotherapeutic process if appropriate reading materials are not available.

The following quote by Zaccaria and Moses (1968) in their classic work on bibliotherapy notes that reading preferences, both individual and general, provide one final guiding principle for using bibliotherapy in the treatment process:

> Reading preferences of children and adolescents go through a series of predictable stages. From the ages of two or three to about six or seven, children like to have stories read to them concerning familiar events. Then up to the age of ten or eleven years, there is an increasing interest in fantasy stories. Adolescents, too, go through several reading stages. The early adolescent (12-15 years) tends to be interested in . . . animal stories, adventure stories, mystery stories, tales of the supernatural, sports stories. . . . Later on (15-18 years) reading preferences change to such topics as war stories, romance, and stories of adolescent life. Perhaps sparked by the realization that maturity is fast approaching, the reading interests in late adolescence (18-21) tend to focus on such types of stories as those that deal with personal values, social significance, strange and unusual human experiences, and the transition to adult life. (p. 102)

THE PROCESS OF BIBLIOTHERAPY

The first step for using bibliotherapy with children is to match the appropriate book or books with the child's presenting problem. Carefully choosing literature will help a child see the similarities between the child's problem and the problem characters are experiencing in a book. The family health practitioner's role at this stage is to help the child develop insight into these similarities.

The child's age determines the depth of what is experienced emotionally by the child in the second stage of the bibliotherapeutic process. With an older child, identification with a book character may lead to an emotional release once the problem is better understood. The clinician can then attempt to guide the older child to insight about and resolution of a presenting problem. Younger children may not be developmentally capable of experiencing an emotional release once a presenting problem is better understood. However, bibliotherapy does allow younger children to see solutions to problems without the use of in-depth verbalization, confrontation, and other strategies often critical to clinical intervention (Pardeck, 1998). With the help of the clinician, younger children can be assisted in identifying with a book character with a problem similar to their own. This process helps children see how a book character solved a presenting problem, and this information may help younger children solve problems confronting them.

Younger children have limited vocabularies, experiences, and short attention spans. Clinicians choosing books for bibliotherapy should carefully consider these kinds of important developmental issues. Arbuthnot and Sutherland (1972) conclude that reading aloud to younger children may help them understand and sympathize with the plights of fictional characters. The therapist, by reading a book aloud, can add emotion and imagery to a book that may not be possible if the child simply reads the book. The process of reading a book aloud may also help facilitate trust between the child and practitioner.

Whipple (1969) notes that books with many illustrations can also facilitate the bibliotherapeutic process with younger children. Illustrations in books often have a positive appeal for children. The greater the number of illustrations in a book, the more likely it is that children will be interested in a story. Whipple suggests that book illustrations in several colors have a greater appeal to younger children than do black-and-white images. Cianciolo (1972) concludes that book illustrations extend the world of children and help them to see that their feelings, wishes, and actions are often part of the normal growth and development process. Animal characters in book illustrations can be particularly useful for helping young children identify with story characters (Pardeck, 1998).

Pardeck (1998) offers the following guidelines that will assist the family health practitioner in book selection for younger children. The books should have appealing illustrations including photographs and pictures. The story content should be interesting to the child. The child should easily understand the book. Books with humor can help maintain a child's interest. Identifying books with surprise, suspense, and recurring refrains should facilitate the bibliotherapeutic process because they help to hold a child's interest.

The Application of the Bibliotherapeutic Process

After book selection, the family health practitioner must decide how to use the book or books in treatment. A critical role of the practitioner is to involve the child in the story situation. This includes encouraging active participation by the child through motor activities, cognitive tasks, and verbalizing reactions to the book. The following points are designed to help the practitioner involve the child in treatment.

- *Reading aloud:* Even though many young children are able to read, most children can benefit from the practitioner's reading a book aloud. By reading aloud, it is much easier to keep a child's attention and interest. By familiarizing oneself with the book before reading it aloud, a practitioner can give more attention to personality traits of book characters, as well as phrases and illustrations that can help the child better identify with book situations and characters. Furthermore, the practitioner may wish to first read a book aloud to himself or herself; this will help the practitioner use the correct pitch, voice tone, and reading pace during critical parts of a story.
- *Observing responses and reactions:* When children are read to they often exhibit many different kinds of important reactions. Some children become emotionally involved in a story. Others may criticize or encourage story characters to behave in a differ-

ent way. Children will also feel anger, joy, envy, and relief as they hear a story read. These are the kinds of responses and reactions that the clinician should attempt to keep track of because they help provide insight into the problems and concerns of children.

- *Follow-up activities:* Many times follow-up activities after a book has been read aloud may not even be needed. Carefully selected books when read aloud will often trigger numerous reactions, including comments and various nonverbal reactions. However, some children may need to be encouraged to respond to a story. The following strategies are suggested:

1. The family health practitioner may have a group of children role-play a different ending to a book.
2. A child may be encouraged to construct a collage or mobile that depicts events in a book.
3. The use of puppets can help a child express feelings about characters and events in a story.
4. Written responses to a story are useful for older children; however, younger children can also benefit from such an activity.
5. A child may be encouraged to dictate how he or she feels about a story character or situation.
6. The practitioner may wish to have the child write a letter to a story character or create a different ending to a story.

These are just a few suggestions for follow-up activities. For a more detailed discussion, see Pardeck (1998).

Using Bibliotherapy with Children of Divorce

Numerous authors have conducted studies on the reaction of children to divorce. For example, Wallerstein and Kelly (1980) found divorce had a significant impact on child development. Kelly (1993) reports that children's reactions to marital separation and divorce can, for some children, be similar to the death of a loved one. Ericson and Tarver-Behring (1999) conclude that if divorcing parents have high conflict or poor communication, it is more likely that children will experience difficulties that interrupt or even cause regression in the normal child development cycle. Conversely, children will be more apt to have minor disruption in their social and emotional development if parents can resolve their differences and issues related to living arrangements in a positive manner (Ericson and Tarver-Behring, 1999). Ericson and Tarver-Behring (1999) summarize the problems associated with divorce as follows:

1. Sadness, grief, loneliness, or depression over the loss of familiar family relationships
2. Anger directed at parents
3. Lowered self-esteem
4. Conflicting loyalties regarding the parents
5. Anxiety about meeting basic needs and a fear of being abandoned
6. Withdrawal from social activities and friends
7. Denial that the divorce has occurred
8. Self-blame or guilt at being the cause of the divorce

Books for Children of Divorce

Many excellent children's books can help the family health practitioner treat children of divorce. The following offers four examples of books that practitioners may find particularly useful for helping young children deal with problems surrounding separation and divorce (Joshua and DiMenna, 2000). These books not only focus on the psychological aspects confronting children of divorce but also stress social environmental issues. This kind of content is critical when applying social intervention based on the family health perspective.

Brown, L. K. and Brown, M. (1988). *Dinosaurs' Divorce: A Guide for Changing Families.* Boston, MA: Little, Brown and Company.

This story stresses that children should not blame themselves when their parents divorce. Parents divorce each other, not their children. The authors also point out that children often feel sad, angry, afraid, guilty, and even ashamed when their parents divorce. Through the use of dinosaurs, this book talks to children about why parents separate and divorce, how to handle visitation, and how to express feelings of hurt when parents divorce. The story is designed for children five to ten years of age and provides a number of clinical insights for children. One insight is that divorce can bring positive changes, another is that children may feel uncomfortable when visiting the parent they used to live with, and last, the child may have to be given permission to love both parents.

Girard, L. W. and Friedman, J. (1991). *At Daddy's on Saturdays*. Morton Grove, IL: Albert Whitman.

This book is about a young girl named Katie whose father moved out of the house after he divorced Katie's mother. Katie is sad and is afraid that her father will not come back to see her. Katie discovers that her father will visit her on a regular basis and that he still loves her. This book is for children ages five to ten. The story offers a number of important clinical insights that may help children of divorce and includes the important point that parents divorce each other and not their children. The authors also stress that children need permission to express all of their feelings. Finally, even though it is hard for children to say good-bye to a parent each week after visits, children discover that their parents continue to love them even though they do not live with them full-time.

Rogers, F. (1996). *Let's Talk About It: Divorce*. New York: Penguin Putnam.

Mr. Rogers speaks to children of divorce about their feelings. These include feelings of sadness, grief, and loneliness. He offers support for children who are feeling the many emotions associated with family breakdown. Mr. Rogers emphasizes ways that children can deal with these feelings. The book is designed for children four to nine years of age. It offers a number of clinical insights that include children's concerns about the parent who has left home, the anxiety they feel concerning who will take care of them, and the importance of children hearing that they did not cause the divorce.

Thomas, S. and Rankin, D. (1997). *Divorced but Still My Parents*. Longmont, CO: Springboard.

This book stresses that some children experience a number of stages as a result of divorce, including denial, anger, bargaining, depression, and acceptance. The authors suggest that some children cannot achieve acceptance of their parents' divorce without working through these stages. They emphasize that this book is most effective when read aloud to children. The book is designed for children six to ten years of age. The authors suggest that not all children experience the stages described in the book. The book is designed for children who appear to be reacting to the separation and divorce of their parents with feelings of loss and confusion. The book offers clinical insights such as children do not cause divorce; divorce means change, but parents still love their children; some kids have one parent; and finally, even when a parent does not see his or her children as often as he or she used to, the absent parent still loves the child.

Case Example

Larry, an eight-year-old boy, is confronted with the divorce of his parents. He knew his parents were having problems because he often heard them arguing after he went to bed. A teacher was one of the first persons to recognize that Larry was having some kind of problem outside the classroom. His grades were falling, homework was never done on time, and he seemed to be withdrawing from activities inside and outside the classroom. The teacher arranged a conference with Larry's parents and discovered that they were divorcing. His parents were not aware that Larry was having problems in school, and they decided he needed professional help.

When Larry began treatment, the practitioner found that he was extremely depressed and angry with his parents for divorcing. Larry, like many children of divorce, felt he was going to be abandoned by his parents and that he was the cause of the divorce. The practitioner designed and implemented a treatment plan that would help Larry focus on these negative feelings. Since Larry was also an extremely bright child and enjoyed reading, the practitioner recommended that Larry read two books about divorce between the first two treatment sessions. These were *Let's Talk About it: Divorce* by Rogers (1996) and *Divorced but Still My Parents* by Thomas and Rankin (1997).

Let's Talk About it: Divorce by Fred Rogers (1996) offered Larry examples of the feelings that children typically have when their parents divorce. Specifically, Larry discovered that children often feel anxiety about their future and worry about who will care for them after their parents break up. *Divorced but Still My Parents* by Shirley Thomas and Dorothy Rankin (1997) helped Larry to better understand the anger, depression, and other negative feelings he was experiencing because of the divorce.

After Larry read the two books, the practitioner encouraged Larry to write down his feelings about what he had read. The practitioner instructed Larry to bring the paper with him to the next treatment session. When the session began, the practitioner encouraged Larry to talk about what he had written. This process helped Larry express his feelings about the divorce. Larry also began to discover that other children who experienced the breakup of their families often felt the emotions he was feeling. In other words, the books helped Larry discover that he was not alone, and that his parents will always love him even though they will now be apart. The practitioner concluded that Larry benefited from reading the two titles and that this reading enhanced the treatment process.

CONCLUSION

Practitioners and researchers have recognized the value of bibliotherapy for helping children cope with various emotional problems and developmental changes (Pardeck, 1998). By providing children with books for dealing with various presenting problems, the family health practitioner can help children (1) gain insight into a problem, (2) focus attention outside the self, (3) realize that they are not alone with a problem, and (4) share their problem with others. Whether the family health practitioner uses bibliotherapy with individual children or with groups of children, books can aid in the exploration and resolution of problems.

One of the most important aspects of using books in treatment is book selection. A number of strategies have been suggested for assisting practitioners in book selection. One final point critical to the effective use of books in treatment is that bibliotherapy is only an adjunct to other forms of intervention; it should never be used as the sole form of treatment.

Bibliotherapy cannot be used with all children, but it certainly can benefit some children. As true of any intervention modality, practitioners need to use sound judgment when using bibliotherapy with children. This chapter has provided guidelines for implementing bibliotherapy successfully and recommended a number of books that practitioners may find useful for helping children deal with the transitions they experience in family life.

REFERENCES

Arbuthnot, M. and Sutherland, Z. (1972). *Children and books*, Fourth edition. Glenview, IL: Foresman.

Cianciolo, P. (1972). What can illustrations offer? In V. M. Read (Ed.), *Reading ladders for human relations*, Fifth edition (pp. 85-119). Washington, DC: American Council on Education.

Ericson, B. O. and Tarver-Behring, S. (1999). When divorce comes to class. In J. F. Kaywell (Ed.), *Using literature to help troubled teenagers cope with family issues* (pp. 120-142). Westport, CT: Greenwood.

Germain, C. (1979). *Social work practice: People and environments*. New York: Columbia University Press.

Goldenberg, I. and Goldenberg, H. (2000). *Family therapy: An overview*, Fifth edition. Belmont, CA: Brooks/Cole.

Goldstein, J., Freud, A., and Solnit, A. J. (1973). *Beyond the best interests of the child*. New York: The Free Press.

Joshua, J. M. and DiMenna, D. (2000). *Read two books and let's talk next week: Using bibliotherapy in clinical practice*. New York: John Wiley.

Kelly, J. (1993). Current research on children's post-divorce adjustment: No simple answers. *Family and Conciliation Courts Review*, 31(1), 29-49.

Minuchin, S. (1974). *Families and family therapy*. Boston: Harvard University Press.

Pardeck, J. T. (1998). *Using books in clinical social work practice: A guide to bibliotherapy*. Binghamton, NY: The Haworth Press.

Pardeck, J. T. and Yuen, F. K. O. (1999). *Family health: A holistic approach to social work practice*. Westport, CT: Auburn House.

Rubin, R. (1978). *Using bibliotherapy: A guide to theory and practice*. Phoenix, AZ: Oryx Press.

Wallerstein, J. S. and Kelly, J. B. (1980). *Surviving the breakup: How children and parents cope with divorce*. New York: Basic Books.

Watson, J. (1980). Bibliotherapy with abused children. *School Counselor*, 27, 204-208.

Whipple, G. (1969). Practical problems of school selection for disadvantaged pupils. In J. Figurel (Ed.), *Reading and realism: Proceedings of the 13th Annual Convention of the International Reading Association* (pp. 195-196). Newark, DE: International Reading Association.

Zaccaria, J. and Moses, H. (1968). *Facilitating human development through reading: The use of bibliotherapy in teaching and counseling*. Champaign, IL: Stipes.

Chapter 4

Adaptive Strategies for Rural Families Living with HIV/AIDS

Susan C. Dollar

INTRODUCTION

Patterns of HIV infection indicate that the spread of the AIDS epidemic into rural areas in America is rising (Centers for Disease Control and Prevention [CDC], 1995). *Rural* is defined as counties outside the boundaries of metropolitan areas with no cities with more than 50,000 residents (Ricketts, Johnson-Webb, and Taylor, 1998). According to figures provided by The National Commission on AIDS (NCOA), the number of AIDS cases swelled in one year (1989) by 37 percent in rural areas while the increase in urban areas remained at 5 percent (NCOA, 1990). Another study of AIDS cases in all U.S. counties reported that most of the top twenty-five counties experiencing rapid increases in AIDS cases were predominantly rural (Lam and Liu, 1994). The Centers for Disease Control and Prevention estimated that 17,170 rural residents were living with AIDS in 1997, and 41,000 to 57,000 rural residents were living with asymptomatic or symptomatic HIV infection (CDC, 1999)

It is important to consider the demographic characteristics of an area when defining it as rural since there is great variance among rural communities. A number of issues that are unique to the rural environment are of concern to providers when dealing with HIV/AIDS clients.

In comparison to their urban counterparts, HIV-infected rural persons experience a more limited access to medical and mental health care, more difficulty coping with life stressors, less access to transportation, more incidents of AIDS-related discrimination, privacy concerns, less satisfaction with life, and greater poverty (Frazier and

Gabel, 1996; Rural Center for AIDS/STD Prevention [RCAP], 2001a). In addition, new medical treatments, comprehensive case-management approaches, and innovative prevention strategies that address the HIV/AIDS epidemic have yet to be adopted in many rural-based health and social service agencies (RCAP, 1994). Although these barriers can hinder service provision, they can be overcome to some extent by recognizing the area's history, norms, and strengths. One of the major strengths of the rural community is its focus on the family unit as the primary support system. An agency would also want to work from an ecological approach, which emphasizes the fit between individuals' adaptive capacities and environmental conditions, and views the community as an important system when seeking solutions (Irey, 1980).

This chapter provides an overview of the HIV epidemic in rural communities and how it affects the individual and his or her family members. Health promotion and disease prevention will be examined within a family health perspective that takes into account the economic, physical, emotional, mental, social, cultural, and spiritual dimensions of family functioning. This conceptual framework provides a holistic view of family needs and suggests areas for interventions to improve family adjustment and well-being during times of crisis (Yuen and Pardeck, 1999).

HIV/AIDS IN THE RURAL CONTEXT

Increasing rates of HIV/AIDS transmission in rural areas can be accounted for by an increase in transmission within rural areas and the migration of persons with HIV infection into rural areas (Berry, 1993; Cohen et al., 1994; Davis and Stapleton, 1991; Rumby et al., 1991). Much of the increase is due to HIV-positive patients returning home to receive care from their families (Berry, 1993; Frazier and Gabel, 1996).

High-Risk Groups

Statistics indicate that heterosexuals, particularly women, as well as people between the ages of 15 and 29 and persons of color are at high risk for HIV transmission in rural areas (RCAP, 1996; Rosenberg, 1995; Rumby et al., 1991). The number of women living with HIV/

AIDS nearly tripled between 1985 and 1994, and 77 percent of these women were Latina or black. In 1999, 44 percent of new HIV infections were among twenty- to twenty-four-year-old women (AIDS Alliance for Children, Youth, and Families, 2000). HIV infection rates are climbing for rural non-Hispanic blacks and Hispanics. A 1995 study estimated "rates of HIV infection to be as high as 2.29 percent among Black males, as low as .05 among White females, and to an average .47 percent for the entire population" (RCAP, 1996, p. 1).

HIV-infected rural residents and their families confront many complex stressors that reduce their overall life quality (Berry, McKinney, and McClain, 1996; Heckman et al., 1998; Rounds, 1988). The stressors are compounded by poverty, a significant factor in the spread and impact of HIV/AIDS in the United States.

Poverty's Impact on HIV/AIDS

Poverty remains a major factor in the spread of HIV/AIDS among rural families. The majority lack essential information and services that would prevent the spread or reduce the impact of HIV disease (Lyons, 2000). The hardest hit populations are African Americans and Hispanics; 30 percent of African Americans and 34 percent of Hispanic Americans live below poverty level in rural areas (Gonzales, 1996). Female-headed, single-parent families are also at a compound risk for HIV/AIDS transmission and exacerbated stressors, as every subgroup of the population—including whites, blacks, Native Americans, and Hispanics—has a significant percentage of the families living below the poverty line (Gonzales, 1996).

The most predominant factors in accounting for the spread of HIV/ AIDS in impoverished rural areas include low educational achievement, fewer financial resources, lack of medical facilities and services (Lyons, 2000; Wodrich et al., 1999), and generally higher rates of chronic disease and mortality (CDC, 1995). Finding adequate and accessible health care and social services for HIV-infected persons is of particular concern in rural areas. Barriers to treatment include lack of health professionals with expertise in infectious disease management; lack of adequate health insurance; and limited support services including transportation, home health care, and hospice and counseling services (RCAP, 1994).

Physical Impact of HIV/AIDS

One of the most difficult obstacles facing families is witnessing the physical suffering of their loved one throughout the disease process. Multiple drug developments have prolonged the life expectancy of HIV-positive individuals, and it has become a manageable chronic condition for many people, but with negative physical side effects. In the initial stages of HIV/AIDS, no signs of physical impairment may appear, and many continue normal life activities. In the later stages, however, when HIV becomes AIDS, there is a wasting away of the body's vital functions and a progressive emaciation caused by the depletion of white blood cells which fight infection. Individuals are susceptible to pneumonia, thrush, herpes, nervous system disorders, and tuberculosis because of immune system breakdown (Kastenbaum, 1991). Families face significant stress in dealing with the later chronic symptoms of the disease and may find it difficult to maintain the stringent medication regimen and make the necessary dietary changes to combat weight loss. There is also stress involved in finding adequate home care and respite care.

Mental and Emotional Impact of HIV/AIDS

The psychological impact of HIV/AIDS on the family is significant and may become insurmountable when family members are not provided with the necessary support. Families are forced to deal with an array of feelings when confronting the terminal disease, including anger, guilt, and shame; fear of contagion; and dealing with family and community rejection when the disease is disclosed to others (AIDS in the Family, 1998). Problems may arise when the infected individual becomes depressed due to declining health, and family members may find it difficult to help the individual comply with treatment and medication regimens (Montaner et al., 1998). In addition, suicide rates are often high among infected individuals as they find it difficult to cope with their declining health (Taylor and Amodei, 1996).

As a consequence of rising HIV infection rates among women of childbearing age, research shows an increase in the number of children being affected by the death of a parent due to the disease (Child Welfare League of America, 1998). In the year 2000, the number of children and adolescents in the United States who will have lost their parents to AIDS was expected to reach between 82,000 and 125,000 (Levine, 1995). For parents who are HIV positive, the task of caregiving for self and children becomes a problem (Hackl, Somlai, and Kalichman, 1997; Kaplan, Marks, and Mertens, 1997; Katz, 1997). Concerns about the disruption in the parenting relationship and the losses they and their children will experience can lead to feelings of grief and loss as well as anger and frustration about how to cope with the future (Hackl, Somlai, and Kalichman, 1997). One qualitative study of HIV-positive women reported that some mothers disengaged from their children to avoid dealing with the inevitable loss and to prepare their children for future independence (Hendrixson, 1997). Further research examining the mental health needs of HIV-positive women found that their stressors concern their children and caretaking roles; social support needs; concerns about death, dying, and despair; and the need for HIV/AIDS information (Hackl, Somlai, and Kalichman, 1997).

Added responsibilities to prepare for the future care of children become a major concern for parents. Consideration of guardianship or adoption for single parents—particularly among those with undocumented immigration status or for those who lack funds for and access to legal counsel—can complicate planning efforts (Antle et al., 2001; Sherr et al, 1993).

Social Impact of HIV/AIDS

Social forces provide some of the largest stressors for the family unit to overcome. According to one study, persons living with HIV/AIDS in a rural Midwestern region struggled with significant social stressors, including a lower satisfaction with life, lower perceptions of social support from family members and friends, and more community stigma and AIDS-related discrimination (Heckman et al., 1998). Traditional moral values and conformity to community norms in many rural communities may account for more stigmatization of people with AIDS, homosexuals, minorities, and drug users, and make effective HIV prevention and outreach difficult (NCOA, 1992).

One of the biggest obstacles to overcome is the perceived and actual prejudice and discrimination against those living with HIV/AIDS and their families (NCOA, 1990). Families face possible isolation and discrimination from friends and extended family due to their member's HIV status. This might include loss of jobs due to stigmatization and declining health, loss of spouse, exclusion from religious or other associations, school dismissal, eviction from household, and fear that children will be taken away (AIDS in the Family, 1998; Hendrixson, 1997). The diagnosis and disclosure of HIV/AIDS contraction within the system greatly impact families. Often, family members and friends socially abandon and reject those who are open about their diagnosis because of the stigma and fear of contagion associated with HIV and its transmission (Barroso, 1997). The individual and family may lose friends and social networks as they are ostracized from their jobs, schools, and churches (AIDS in the Family, 1998).

For HIV-positive men who have sex with men, rural areas present many threats, which leaves them feeling isolated and disenfranchised. Many remained secretive about their sexual orientation before being diagnosed HIV positive, but after diagnosis they must contend with disclosure of not only the illness but also their same-sex orientation. Whereas the family of origin is usually the primary social support for persons experiencing the crisis of an illness, this support is not always available for gay men with HIV/AIDS due to homophobia and the stigma associated with AIDS (Kadushin, 1996).

Another social stressor is the perceived or actual lack of anonymity and confidentiality, which may be experienced in rural areas when seeking health or support services (Frazier and Gabel, 1996). Fear of being ostracized for being HIV positive can force people to seek drug treatment or medical assistance in urban areas, or prevent them from being tested and discussing sexual practices with clinicians. They may also isolate themselves from other support mechanisms (RCAP, 1994).

Cultural and Spiritual Stressors

Cultural beliefs may influence the decision to seek treatment for HIV-positive individuals and their families. For communities of color, mistrust of the legal system due to immigration status, fear of racism, or fear that they will lose custody of their children may prevent early diagnosis and treatment (Siegel and Gorey, 1994). Cultural beliefs may also influence a mother's choice in making formal guardianship arrangements when facing imminent death due to HIV/AIDS. Often, women of color will expect their family members to care for their children after their death (Groce, 1995)

Spiritual dimensions of the family may be directly challenged during the course of the individual's illness. The infected individual and his or her family members typically face the stages of dealing with death, which may bring about a renewed sense of responsibility, meaning, and purpose in life (Hendrixson, 1997). Many cope with the disease by improving the communication and the quality of life they share with others in order to leave family members with positive images of the infected individual (Antle et al., 2001). In one study of women living with HIV, some reported positive self-esteem changes and a growing sense of empowerment as time progressed (Hendrixson, 1997). Others may face their terminal disease with fear, guilt, and bitterness, which can damage the spiritual relationship if they believe in a higher power (McDaniel, Hepworth, and Doherty, 1997).

FAMILY AND COMMUNITY INTERVENTIONS

Management of the HIV/AIDS epidemic in rural areas requires a diverse and coordinated response by local, regional, and national leadership. Often, urban models for service delivery and prevention education are inappropriate to rural areas (RCAP, 1994). Successful approaches have been developed that focus on increasing the ability of families and communities to care for those who are HIV/AIDS infected. The next section describes some of these strategies.

Building Family Supports

A family health perspective is important to improving the overall quality of life and well-being of persons living with HIV/AIDS. This is particularly important in rural areas where the family is the primary caregiver and a major source of social support for the infected individual (Taylor and Amodei, 1996). A family systems perspective involves including family members and significant others in the helping process and considering the family as a whole when designing treatment and prevention programs (Yuen and Pardeck, 1999).

Several family-centered interventions are recommended for improving adaptive skills and coping responses. Interventions to help family members control and understand the psychological and emotional problems of HIV/AIDS—such as anxiety, depression, feelings of interpersonal sensitivity, and anger—will improve functioning and well-being (McShane, Bumbalo, and Patsdaughter, 1994). Interventions may include individual, family, or group counseling, the latter perhaps requiring travel to the nearest city. Support groups can be instrumental in helping families participate in activities that improve communication skills and health-promotion behaviors, such as relaxation techniques, hobbies, dietary changes, rest, and exercise (Antle et al., 2001; RCAP, 2001b). In addition, farm families have historically demonstrated great resilience and self-reliance, and social workers should build upon the family's existing strengths to improve the coping abilities. Identifying past family successes during crises, recognizing effective coping strategies, and addressing limitations within the family system are a large part of how the family can begin to normalize reaction to the disease (Greif and Porembski, 1988). Communication skills should be practiced in order for the family to confront difficult issues together, such as death and dying, child custody, financial issues (Kadushin, 1996), or homosexuality of an HIV-infected family member (Landau-Stanton and Clements, 1993).

The family health perspective would also prescribe educating the family about the physical dimensions of the disease, thereby reducing the fear, dependence, and shame associated with HIV/AIDS. Caregivers should provide information on self-protection, modes of HIV transmission, treatment, and the course of the disease (Frierson, Lippmann, and Johnson, 1987; Lovejoy, 1990). Many family members need hope regarding the prognosis. Information about new pharmacotherapies that extend life and prolong health can help (Britton and Zarski, 1989). Finally, information and referral concerning medical treatment, long-term care, and social service support is important in instilling hope and activating problem solving within the family unit (Faulstich, 1987; Frierson, Lippmann, and Johnson, 1987). Support groups are extremely important in helping family members buffer against stress and for increasing coping resources by discussing concerns with others, asking questions, and receiving mutual-support (Goggin et al., 2001; Lyons, 2000).

Building Social Support in the Community

The family health perspective requires an ecosystem intervention package that includes organizational and community-level changes that will facilitate long-range improvements in the rural community's infrastructure. Perhaps the most difficult element of change is effectively reaching an audience and changing its attitudes and perceptions about HIV/AIDS. HIV-prevention education and social action to improve or expand services should be sensitively designed with an understanding of the community's values and traditions. Having trusted health professionals or civic leaders from the immediate or surrounding region provide factual information about HIV/AIDS is likely to be more successful than inviting outside experts or providing personal testimonials from strangers.

Improved access to health care is repeatedly mentioned in the literature as a vital need in rural communities (Heckman et al., 1998). Rural HIV-positive individuals who seek health and social services must overcome a host of barriers to participation, such as vast geographic distances between practitioners and clients, limited transportation, and physical disabilities that preclude many HIV-infected rural persons from traveling to face-to-face support services. In addition, heightened concerns regarding confidentiality prevent many HIV-infected rural persons from attending mental-health support services.

To improve access to care, medical services, prevention activities, financial services, and social services must be integrated through collaborative arrangements established between agencies. Case management should be employed to deliver a coordinated system of comprehensive care for patients and to reduce duplication of services. Leveraging limited resources between public and private partnerships improves the capacity of the community to care for those with HIV/AIDS and their families (RCAP, 2001a). Health care personnel shortages and the lack of medical information can be addressed by expanding telemedicine technologies to help diagnose and treat HIV/AIDS, as well as increasing use of videos and informational Web sites to expand support and information concerning the disease and available resources (RCAP, 2001a).

Alternative services that are consistent with cultural mores or evolving cultural adaptation should also be considered by rural communities to expand their capacity to care for the HIV/AIDS community and their families when using the family health perspective. Assisting kinship networks to provide care is one such alternative. Providing community support, whether financial or social, enables the family to remain intact and functional during crises. Home care, hospice care, and child care for AIDS patients and their families meet an immediate need for support through volunteers at local civic, school, and church organizations. Other improvements include protecting at-risk children and youth by providing alternative education options, school drop-out prevention, tutoring, after-school drop-in centers, child care for young parents, sports and recreation, peer drug counseling, education and prevention, skills training for older children, and establishing organizations for children (Antle et al., 2001; Lyons, 2000).

Churches and other religious organizations have been an influential force in rural areas by providing financial, social, and emotional support for community members. Innovative outreach programs, including food pantries, transportation services, respite care, and home visits, have been established in many areas to fill a service gap in some communities. Rural residents often view these services with less stigma than publicly funded programs, and a broader constituency consequently accesses the services.

Finally, and perhaps most importantly, is the need for primary and secondary prevention within the community, aimed particularly at at-risk groups. A society's reluctance to accept and deal with the disease in their communities is partially the result of a lack of accurate information regarding the disease, how it is transmitted, and treatment alternatives (RCAP, 1994). Prevention and treatment education will also help to reduce discrimination against and enhance tolerance for people living with HIV/AIDS.

A Case Study Example: The Ruiz Family Works Through a Family Crisis

This case study illustrates how a family health perspective based on an ecological approach can help persons with HIV/AIDS and their families cope with the disease.

The Agency System

A case manager at a community-based AIDS agency in a rural farming community addresses basic income, medical and emergency housing as well as palliative care for those in the latter stages of AIDS. The agency has two volunteers that assist with transportation for clients who are ill or without transportation to appointments. This agency is the only one in the community that provides prevention and treatment services for HIV-infected/affected individuals, and according to a recent survey conducted by the agency, many in the community do not know how HIV is transmitted and hold many misconceptions about who can become infected by HIV/AIDS and how it can be medically treated.

The Client System

Carla Ruiz is a forty-eight-year-old Hispanic female diagnosed as HIV positive. She arrived as a walk-in client, explaining that, following her diagnosis, she had moved back to her hometown after leaving her job and husband. Carla suspects that she contracted HIV from her husband, Ray, who admitted to having extramarital affairs and unprotected sex. He has been told about her diagnosis and is currently being tested for the virus. With little savings, she and her two young sons moved in with her parents. She told her parents and sister, who live in the same town, about her illness, but she has not talked to her children about her illness. The immediate family is supportive of Carla and her children and has assured her that they will be there for her by providing shelter, food, and emotional support until she can get back on her feet. Carla appears in good spirits despite her recent diagnosis and wants assistance with finding work, medical care, and enrolling the children in school.

The Intervention Strategy

Family health interventions in this case should involve individual, family, group, and community responses. The first meeting should involve a family assessment including family composition, family genogram, family strengths and challenges, and planning for services. Some of the most important work is in the initial interview with Carla and her immediate family. Ensure privacy for the family and work through a list of priorities for Carla and her family using the seven family health dimensions (physical, economic, mental, emotional, social, cultural, and spiritual). Carla states that immediate medical attention and a Medicaid referral to the county hospital is arranged along with transportation. Both she and her family need financial and emotional support. The social worker should stress to the family the importance of maintaining both mental and physical well-being through good nutrition and exercise. Socialization with family and friends should also be encouraged, since Carla's family appears to be close-knit and rely on one another for material and emotional support. Follow up with a home visit to meet extended family members and friends who might serve as a natural support. Educate the family about the disease from a medical, mental, and emotional perspective concerning how to care for someone with HIV, and provide family members with information about informal support groups that may help them deal with caregiver stress.

There is also a concern about enrolling the children in school and the effect the move has had on them. Carla stated that she needs counseling concerning her approach to telling her children and other significant persons about her illness. Suggest to Carla that she talk with the school social worker about her chronic illness when enrolling the children in school so he or she will be prepared to help the children cope with the transition to a new school as well as deal with the eventual realization about their mother's chronic illness.

Cultural and spiritual issues should also be addressed for Carla and her family by providing bilingual/bicultural counseling and information to Spanish-speaking family members. Culturally appropriate spiritual guidance with issues such as death and dying, guilt and shame about her HIV status, and dealing with family conflict surrounding her impending divorce from her husband may be needed. Carla will eventually need to arrange for legal services for adoption care following her death, which can be dealt with through a pro bono attorney referral from the agency. In addition to financial assistance and job placement, the caseworker should talk with Carla about support programs, formal and informal, that could help her with emotional and spiritual support when needed.

After arranging for immediate services and educating the family about the disease process and support programs, address the need for expanding family-centered education in the community. The needs assessment determined that more education is needed in the community to inform others about HIV/AIDS. Schedule a community forum to discuss how churches, social service agencies, university extension, schools, and other community groups may be able to respond to families in crisis. Volunteers to provide HIV outreach services and prevention education in schools and community centers should be identified and trained. The social worker should also suggest a fundraising effort for expanding alternative services, such as respite care and support group for the chronically ill. Conduct a continual community assessment in order to determine if services are appropriate and adequate and if community perceptions of HIV/AIDS have changed as a result of outreach and prevention education efforts.

CONCLUSION

HIV/AIDS has become a serious problem for rural America. Families who live in rural areas experience chronic stressors that are rooted in the many risks associated with rural residence. Rural family needs cannot be addressed in isolation from the condition of the communities in which these families are located. Rural social and economic conditions are diverse, which necessitates developing local initiatives that address the unique nature of the problems confronting these rural families.

New strategies and programs are needed to help HIV-positive individuals and their families cope with difficulties of the disease. One of these strategies is the family health perspective. It is a strategy that is family focused and takes into account the strengths that lie within the family unit and kinship network when dealing with crises. The community must be involved in providing support to families through alternative delivery systems and encouraging public and private partnerships to share resources and introduce or expand needed financial and service care systems. Volunteer efforts should also be expanded to provide care to HIV-positive individuals and their families through support groups, fundraising, and prevention education efforts. Combined, these can change beliefs, attitudes, behavior, and treatment of the disease and will contribute to a reduction in HIV/AIDS transmission in rural communities.

REFERENCES

AIDS Alliance for Children, Youth, and Families (2000). *Reaching Women of Color.* Available online at <www.aids-alliance.org/img/gv2/nonstandard_files/aids_alliance/women_of_color.pdf>.

AIDS in the family: Social and emotional stressors (1998). Available online at <www.seatec.emory.edu/SEATEC/resources/psychosocial/AIDSFamily.pdf>.

Antle, B., Well, L., Goldie, R., Robyn, S., DeMatteo, D., and King, S. (2001). Challenges of parenting for families living with HIV/AIDS. *Social Work, 46*(2), 159-171.

Barroso, J. (1997). Reconstructing my life: Becoming a long-term survivor of AIDS. *Qualitative Health Research, 7*(1), 57-75.

Berry, D. (1993). The emerging epidemiology of rural AIDS. *Journal of Rural Health, 9,* 293.

Berry, D., McKinney, M., and McClain, M. (1996). Rural HIV service networks: Patterns of care and policy issues. *AIDS and Public Policy Journal, 11,* 36-46.

Britton, P. J. and Zarski, J. J. (1989). HIV spectrum disorders and the family: Selected interventions based on stylistic dimensions. *AIDS Care, 1,* 85-92.

Centers for Disease Control and Prevention (CDC) (1995). First 500,000 AIDS cases—United States, 1995. *Morbidity and Mortality Weekly Report, 44*(46), 849-852.

Centers for Disease Control and Prevention (CDC) (1999). *HIV/AIDS Surveillance Supplemental Report, 5*(1), 8.

Child Welfare League of America (1998). Alternative permanency planning: Legal options for HIV-infected parents. *HIV Permanency Planning Newsletter, 2,* 1-7. Available online at <www.cwla.org/programs/hivaids/hivnews2.htm>.

Cohen, S., Klein, J., Mohr, J., van der Horst, C., and Weber, D. (1994). The geography of AIDS: Patterns of urban and rural migration. *Southern Medical Journal, 87*(6), 599-606.

Davis, K. and Stapleton, J. (1991). Migration in rural areas by HIV patients: Impact of HIV-related health care use. *Infection Control Hospital Epidemiology, 12,* 550.

Faulstich, M. E. (1987). Psychiatric aspects of AIDS. *American Journal of Psychiatry, 144,* 551-556.

Frazier, E. M. and Gabel, L. L. (1996). HIV/AIDS in family practice: An approach to care in rural areas. *Family Practice Recertification, 18,* 59-77.

Frierson, R. L., Lippmann, S. B., and Johnson, J. (1987). AIDS: Psychological stresses on the family. *Psychosomatics, 28,* 65-68.

Goggin, K., Catley, D., Briscon, S. T., Engelson, E. S., Rabkin, J. G., and Kotler, D. P. (2001). A female perspective on living with HIV disease. *Health and Social Work, 26*(2), 80-90.

Gonzales, J. L. (1996). *Racial and ethnic groups in America,* Third edition. Dubuque, IA: Kendall/Hunt.

Greif, G. L. and Porembski, E. (1988). AIDS and significant others: Findings from a preliminary exploration of needs. *Health and Social Work, 13,* 259-265.

Groce, N. E. (1995). Children and AIDS in multicultural perspective. In S. Geballe, J. Gruendel, and W. Andiman (Eds.), *Forgotten children of the AIDS epidemic* (pp. 95-106). New Haven, CT: Yale University Press.

Hackl, K. L., Somlai, A. M., and Kalichman, S. C. (1997). Women living with HIV/AIDS: The dual challenge of being a patient and caregiver. *Health and Social Work, 22*(1), 53-63.

Heckman, T. G., Somlai, A., Kalichman, S. C., Franzoi, S. L., and Kelly, J. A. (1998). Psychological differences between urban and rural persons living with HIV/AIDS. *Journal of Rural Health, 14,* 138-146.

Hendrixson, L. L. (1997). The psychological and psychosexual impact of HIV/AIDS disease on rural women: A qualitative study (Doctoral dissertation, New York University, 1996). *Dissertation Abstracts International, 57*(12), 5312A.

Irey, K. V. (1980). The social work generalist in a rural context: An ecological perspective. *Journal of Education for Social Work, 16*(3), 36-42.

Kadushin, G. (1996). Gay men with AIDS and their families of origin: An analysis of social support. *Health and Social Work, 21*(2), 141-150.

Kaplan, M. S., Marks, G., and Mertens, S. B. (1997). Distress and coping among women with HIV infection: Preliminary finding from a multiethnic sample. *American Journal of Orthopsychiatry, 67,* 80-91.

Kastenbaum, R. K. (1991). *Death society and human experience,* Fifth edition. Needham Heights, MA: Allyn & Bacon.

Katz, D. A. (1997). The profile of HIV infection in women: A challenge to the profession. *Social Work in Health Care, 24*(3/4), 127-134.

Lam, N. and Liu, K. (1994). Spread of AIDS in rural America, 1982-1990. *Journal of Acquired Immune Deficiency Syndrome, 7,* 485-490.

Landau-Stanton, J. and Clements, C. (1993). *AIDS health and mental health: A primary sourcebook.* New York: Brunner/Mazel.

Levine, C. (1995). Orphans of the HIV epidemic: Unmet needs in six U.S. cities. *AIDS Care, 7*(Suppl. 1), 557-562.

Lovejoy, N. (1990). AIDS: Impact on the gay man's homosexual and heterosexual families. In E. Bozett and S. Sussman (Eds.), *Homosexuality and family relations* (pp. 285-316). Binghamton, NY: The Haworth Press.

Lyons, M. (2000). The impact of HIV and AIDS on children, families and communities: Risks and realities of childhood during the HIV epidemic. Available online at <www.undp.org/hiv/publications/issues/english/issue30e.html>.

McDaniel, S. H., Hepworth, J., and Doherty, W. J. (1997). *The shared experiences of illness: Stories of patients, families and their therapists.* New York: Harper-Collins.

McShane, R., Bumbalo, J., and Patsdaughter, C. (1994). Psychological distress in family members living with human immunodeficiency virus/acquired immune deficiency syndrome. *Archives of Psychiatric Nursing, 8,* 53-61.

Montaner, J., Reiss, P., Cooper, D., Vella, S., Harris, M., Conway, B., Wainberg, M. A., Smith, D., Robinson, P., Hall, D., et al. (1998). A randomized, double-blind trial comparing combinations of nevirapine, didanosine, and zidovudine for HIV-infected patients: The INCAS trial. *Journal of the American Medical Association, 279,* 930-937.

National Commission on AIDS (1990). *Report number three: Research, the workforce and the HIV epidemic in rural America.* Washington, DC: Author.

National Commission on AIDS (1992). *AIDS in rural America.* Washington, DC: Author.

Ricketts, T., Johnson-Webb, K., and Taylor, P. (1998). *Definitions of rural: A handbook of health policy makers and researchers* (Technical Issues Paper, Federal Office of Rural Health Policy, North Carolina Rural Health Research Program, Cecil G. Sheps Center for Health Services Research). Chapel Hill: University of North Carolina.

Rosenberg, P. S. (1995). Scope of the AIDS epidemic in the United States. *Science, 270,* 1372-1375.

Rounds, K. (1988). AIDS in rural areas: Challenges to providing care. *Social Work, 33,* 257-261.

Rumby, R., Shappley, N., Waivers, L., and Esinhart, J. (1991). AIDS in rural eastern North Carolina. Patient migration: A rural AIDS burden. *AIDS, 5*(11), 1373-1378.

Rural Center for AIDS/STD Prevention (RCAP) (1994). HIV infection and AIDS in rural America. *Rural Prevention Report, 1*(1), 1-7.

Rural Center for AIDS/STD Prevention (RCAP) (1996). HIV/AIDS in rural America. *Fact Sheet, 8*, 1-4.

Rural Center for AIDS/STD Prevention (RCAP) (2001a). Elements of successful HIV prevention efforts identified by CDC. *Rural Prevention Report, 6*(1), 1-4.

Rural Center for AIDS/STD Prevention (RCAP) (2001b). Mental health needs of HIV-infected rural persons. *Fact Sheet, 13*, 1-2.

Sherr, L., Petrak, J., Melvin, D., Davey, T., Glover, L., and Hedge, B. (1993). Psychosocial needs expressed by the natural caregivers of HIV infected children. *AIDS Care, 3*, 331-343.

Siegel, K. and Gorey, E. (1994). Childhood bereavement due to parental death from acquired immunodeficiency syndrome. *Journal of Developmental and Behavioral Pediatrics, 25*, 581-593.

Taylor, E. R. and Amodei, N. (1996). The presence of psychiatric disorders in HIV-infected women. *Journal of Counseling and Development, 74*(4), 345-352. Available online at EBSCOhost database.

Wodrich, D. L., Swerdlik, M. E., Chenneville, T., and Landau, S. (1999). HIV/AIDS among children and adolescents: Implications for the changing role of school psychologists. *School Psychology Review, 28*(2), 228-242. Available online at EBSCOhost database.

Yuen, F. and Pardeck, J. T. (1999). Family health: A family health approach to social work practice. In J. T. Pardeck and F. Yuen (Eds.), *A holistic approach to social work practice* (pp. 1-16.). Westport CT: Auburn House.

Chapter 5

Beyond Crisis Intervention: Services for Families with Children with Disabilities

Ute C. Orgassa

INTRODUCTION

Families exist in a great variety and complexity. However, certain basic elements are alike, such as the identity of the family versus the outside world and the attempt by family members to deal with crises within the boundaries of the family unit first. The way a family copes in a crisis situation is shaped by its unique circumstances and challenges. Life-altering events and crises can happen to every family at any time. Service providers need to be able to help families through life crises. The crisis discussed here is the realization that one family member has a disability.

Family health social work practice (Pardeck et al., 1998; Pardeck and Yuen, 1997, 1999; Yuen, Skibinski, and Pardeck, 2003) proposes a holistic approach to social work with families. Within their unique eco-systems, families with children with disabilities encounter particular stresses and challenges. Different families have their own meanings for and interpretations of the disabilities, develop specific coping strategies, and have different needs. Family health social workers employ a variety of service technologies to assist these families and children.

FAMILIES WITH CHILDREN WITH DISABILITIES

Families with children with disabilities live in a different crisis situation than other families because their problems are both acute situational crisis events and developmental events. Therefore, they need both immediate and long-term services that help them cope with a different reality. The families face many stressors that are unique to their situation. Those stressors are added to the everyday strains that typical families encounter. One of the daily stressors that families with children with disabilities face is the physical care necessary for the child to function, which does not change in the amount of tasks and may become only more strenuous over the years as the child grows. Many stressors are clearly tied to transitions in the life cycle, such as the transitions from home to school, school to work, or other work-related settings.

However, to understand the unique situation in which families with children with disabilities live, one has to look at the beginning of the experience—the first acute crisis situation they face—which is the discovery of the child's disability. The way a family copes with this first crisis profoundly influences their ability to face the challenges that follow.

The Discovery of Disability

A disability can be discovered at many different points in a child's life. For some, it can be discovered before the birth of the child due to prenatal screenings or an ultrasound that showed an anomaly. For other parents, the disability is detected at birth or very shortly thereafter. As with parents who face a disability before birth, these parents learn that their child is different. The extent of the disability is usually unknown at this time, and parents are left with many unknowns.

For some parents the realization that their child has a disability, or is different from other children, is a gradual process that takes much observation and convincing of medical authorities that something is wrong. Adoptive parents may discover that their child has a disability after the adoption.

Regardless of how the disability is discovered, it is a major crisis for the parents because a child with a disability is usually not what they expected. It constitutes a nonnormative event. An event is non-normative when it happens at an unanticipated time or has a different outcome than expected (McCubbin and Figley, 1983). Suddenly they are different from other people and have to adjust their dreams, knowledge, and expectations to the new situation. An exception to this is the family who knowingly adopts a child with a disability.

THE DOUBLE ABCX MODEL

Once a disability is detected many different factors influence the way a family deals with the situation. To determine a family's options one needs to look at crisis, coping, and stressors in general. First, every family experiences stressors and crises; they are a part of life. Second, the way families handle crises depends strongly on the types of stressful life experiences they had before the new event, on the way the family interacts in general, on if they live in a supportive or nonsupportive environment, and how they perceive their situations.

A model that describes this interaction in detail is the double ABCX model created by McCubbin and Patterson (1983). It is based on the ABCX model by Reuben Hill (1949, 1958). Hill (1949) defined A as the stressor event, B as the resources of the family, C as the appraisal of the situation by the family, and X as the crisis. A crisis can lead to positive as well as negative outcomes for the family, depending on factors A, B, and C.

McCubbin and Patterson (1983) expanded this model because they realized that a crisis or a stressor is not just a one-time event. A stressor does not happen out of context or in a vacuum. Therefore they defined Aa as the stressor-event in addition to the pile-up of other stressors and strains, Bb as the family resources, Cc as the perception of both Aa and Bb by the family, and Xx as the crisis or change of the family that led to either "bonadaptation" or maladaptation, meaning positive or negative adjustment to the new situation.

It is important to understand that stressors (Aa) can be both positive and negative. For example, the birth of a child by itself is a stressor, albeit for many people a positive one. It involves a major life change with many hopes, dreams, and expectations connected to it as well as fear and a feeling of being overwhelmed. Depending on the relationship that existed before the birth of a child can accelerate the deterioration of the parents' relationship or it can strengthen it. Cowan and Cowan (2000) found that by the time children reach eighteen months of age, 12.5 percent of marriages that were deemed stable before the birth ended in divorce or separation.

The resources (Bb) a family has include the way they treat one another as well as the availability of extended family, friends, and professional help. In other words, it includes their coping strategies and formal and informal social support. These resources can differ from what the family perceives (Cc) it has. Two families in an almost identical situation with regard to stressors and resources can have very different outcomes. The family that perceives the stressor as huge and their resources as limited will have a more negative outcome than the family that perceives the stressor as something they can handle and their resources as plentiful.

The crisis itself is what happens when those three factors (Aa, Bb, Cc) are put together. It involves a change of the situation in any case, for better or worse, depending on the individual case.

Coping

The way a family reacts to a crisis is called coping. Coping has several different aspects. Coping concerns the actions as well as the emotions of the family (Lazarus and Folkman, 1984). Coping is a process that includes the entire family and is defined by Pearlin and Turner (1987) as "the things that people do to avoid being harmed by lifestrains" (p. 33). The actions or behaviors that the family members use in this situation are their coping skills.

The Double ABC Factors in Regard to the Family with a Member with a Disability

Stressors Faced Within the Family

Once a child with a disability is born, or a disability is detected, a family faces many challenges. First, the family must come to terms with the changed reality. Then family members have to learn about the different aspects of the disability and the options available for coping with them.

The changed reality may look very different to different family members. For example, mothers tend to concentrate most on the actual caretaking demands that the child with the disability has and will have for a long time. They may grieve their loss of freedom. Fathers may look at the situation from a financial standpoint and worry about medical bills and insurance coverage. Several negative outcomes have been identified in the literature (see Marsh, 1992, for a review) concerning the adjustment of different family members to a child with a disability. For mothers, some concerns can be caregiver burden, lifetime expectations of caregiving, and problems with identity and self-concept (Marsh, 1992). Fathers often experience being regarded as peripheral in raising a child with a disability, or they may withdraw on their own. Feelings of depression, inferiority, and low self-esteem are associated with this. Fathers are also more concerned about the economical burden and the meaning of disability to the outside world (Marsh, 1992). Both parents experience mourning for the expected child (Seligman and Darling, 1997).

The marital relationship can suffer because a child with a disability brings fear, guilt, anger, and fatigue into the relationship in an amount that may not have been present before. Marriages have to be reorganized under these new circumstances, and, depending on the surrounding factors, the relationships may not withstand the strain (Marsh, 1992).

Siblings have to battle with loneliness, anger, guilt, embarrassment, identification, and confusion. They also fear contagion, lifelong responsibility, the possibility of their own children having a disability, and they experience the financial drain on their family (Marsh, 1992).

Grandparents are likely to mourn the loss of an expected grandchild to carry on the family tradition, as well as the reduced opportunities for their children. Grandparents have been found to deny the severity of the disability, to blame the partner of their child for the disability, to search for every available treatment or cure, and to withdraw from the family (Marsh, 1992).

The negative consequences previously listed have to be put into perspective. Not all families experience them and not all families experience them to the same degree. The negative results were such because research focused mostly on the negative consequences of disability on parents and siblings (Seligman and Darling, 1997). The research measured the disability as the most important independent variable and used variables such as depression or marital dysfunction as the dependent variables.

Research also exists that looks at more positive outcomes as well as contributing factors to those outcomes. If the disability is the Aa factor within the double ABCX model, researchers look also at the resources or the Bb factor and the perceptions or the Cc factor for positive aspects.

Researchers have found that there are many more factors influencing bonadaptation or maladaptation than just the disability of the child. Socioeconomic status, gender of the child (Marsh, 1992), religiosity (Pargament, 1990; Leyser, 1994), adaptation before the birth of the child (Herman and Thompson, 1995), social support (Dunst et al., 1990), cultural influences, formal help systems (Levy et al., 1996), and family relations (Bristol, Gallagher, and Schopler, 1988) all influence the way a family copes with this event.

Newer research looks at more cognitive coping strategies (Turnbull et al., 1993). The family's outlook on the situation influences the way members cope much more than the initial situation does (Affleck and Tennen, 1993; Antonovsky, 1993; Brown, 1993; McCubbin et al., 1993). In addition to this, the family structure regarding cohesion and communication makes a big difference (Boss, 1993; Patterson, 1993).

Because of the emphasis on the entire family system, there is as much importance placed on fathers, siblings, and grandparents as there is on mothers (Meyer, 1993). Fathers and siblings are regarded as important components of the family system that influence the adjustment to the disability by the whole family. Fathers and siblings need support systems just as mothers do to effectively cope with the disability and society's reaction to it.

Grandparents are considered, on the one hand, as extended family, and on the other hand as a social support system that can either help tremendously or put additional strain on the family (Glasberg and Harris, 1997; Schilmoeller and Baranowski, 1998).

Parents of children with disabilities who write about their coping strategies also influence the recent literature. Interestingly, parents list their children with disabilities as positive coping factors both in regard to coping with the disability and other family crises (Schulz, 1993; Vohs, 1993). Parents rely on their children with disabilities to help them in life-cycle transitions. They use their children's coping strategies as examples for their own, and parents understand the positive qualities their children bring into their families.

Stressors Outside the Family

Seligman and Darling (1997) list being exposed to stigma as a negative consequence of having a family member with a disability.

Stigma, or the realization that the environment views the family as different from normal, can lead to a desire to be considered very typical in all other aspects of life.

A study that assessed the role relations of families with children with developmental disabilities found that, besides the disability issue, families desired to be as "normal" as possible (Traustadottir, 1995). These families define normal as being that the father provides financial support, and the mother takes care of the disability-related needs of the child and the emotional needs of the family. This can put additional strains on families that have not adhered to conventional role relations before.

Social support can tremendously influence the disability experience as well. Ell (1984) defines social support as "the emotional support, advice, guidance, and appraisal, as well as the material aid and services, that people obtain from their social relationships" (p. 134).

Social support is divided into two categories: informal and formal. Informal social support refers to help from family members, friends, neighbors, acquaintances, colleagues, and the community that is not formally requested and paid for. Formal support involves the service system. Social support is regarded as one of the major factors that influence the well-being of families. Informal support is regarded as very important when it comes to coping (Herman and Thompson, 1995).

For example, if the family has just one friend or extended family member that also has a child with a disability and knows how to navigate the system, they can see that life with a child with a disability is possible and that options are available. It is also said that families with children with disabilities lack informal social support (Levy et al., 1996).

The Service Providers

The formal support system for families can be both a blessing and a burden. Many families with children with disabilities have to meet with numerous medical and nonmedical specialists. For example, Thyer and Kropf (1995) identified fifteen different service providers commonly used by these families. The fifteen did not even include medical specialists, who undoubtedly play a major role in most disability cases. Orgassa (2001) identified twenty-six different service providers for families with children with developmental disabilities. Each one was used by at least some of the families interviewed.

Specialists do not necessarily talk with one another or use similar and understandable terms that are easy for the family to follow. A need exists for the family to make time to visit, understand, and coordinate with all service providers and their perspectives.

This is a very time-consuming and stressful task that can also be disheartening and frustrating. Many medical service providers still operate under a deficit model, so parents will hear many times what their children cannot do or will not be able to do.

SERVICES AND INTERVENTIONS FOR FAMILIES WITH CHILDREN WITH DISABILITIES

Within this challenging service system there is a need for social work practitioners to help families. Social work practitioners meet families with children with disabilities in a variety of settings and functions. Among them are schools, hospitals, income maintenance, child protective services, and advocacy. Families identified social work services as helpful in supplementing their informal support system (Levy et al., 1996; Herman and Marenco, 1997; Honig and Winger, 1997).

Nature of Services

Services that have been regarded as helpful for and by families have some common characteristics. They are family-centered and family-focused (Corrigan and Bishop, 1997; Dempsey, 1996; Marsh, 1992; McBride et al., 1993; Petr, 1998; Trivette et al., 1995), they include informal support systems (Mausner, 1995; Petr, 1994), and they are empowering for the families (Dempsey, 1996; Kalyanpur and Rao, 1991; McCallion and Toseland, 1993).

These characteristics refer more to the "how" of service delivery than to the specific services that are delivered. Services that are delivered in a way that respect families and their decision-making processes, that are more oriented to prevention of crises than to their management, and that include more than just the child and the mother are readily accepted by families and show a greater impact.

Several authors have highlighted the importance of positive encounters with service providers (Alexander and Tomkins-McGill, 1987; Beckman, 1996; Biggs, 1997; Marsh, 1992; McBride et al., 1993; Petr, 1994). Collaboration between service providers and families allows families to see the service provider as part of the solution rather than part of the problem, and ensures that the necessary attention is given by all parties to the problems at hand.

Family-Centered Services

Family-centered services are described by Dunst, Trivette, and Deal (1994); Dunst and collegues (1993); Dunst, Trivette, and Thompson (1990); and Johnson (1990). These services have several characteristics:

1. They recognize that the family is the only constant in regard to service provision. Service providers change over time.
2. They try to facilitate parent/professional collaboration on all levels of care.
3. They honor the racial, ethnic, cultural, and socioeconomic diversity of families.
4. They promote the sharing of unbiased and complete information with parents on an ongoing basis and in an appropriate and supportive manner.
5. They promote the implementation of appropriate policies and programs that are comprehensive and provide emotional and financial support to meet the needs of the families.
6. They recognize family strengths and individuality and respect different methods of coping.
7. They emphasize an understanding of and incorporation of the developmental needs of infants, children, and adolescents.
8. They encourage and facilitate parent-to-parent support and networking.
9. They assure that the service delivery system is flexible, accessible, and responsive to families (adapted from Johnson, 1990, p. 237).

Family-centered services can empower families and support them in ways that neither are threatening nor promote dependence.

The Content of the Services

The specific social services that are considered most important by families are facilitation of respite care (Herman and Thompson, 1995; Lightburn and Pine, 1996; Petr, 1994), counseling (Lightburn and Pine, 1996), location of financial support (Herman and Thompson, 1995), and case management (Levy et al., 1996; McCallion and Toseland, 1993).

Respite care gives parents the time and opportunity to recover from their caregiving duties and to do other things that are important in their lives. Counseling can help all members of the family adjust to complicated issues in their lives—disability related or not. Location of financial support is an important social-work task, because the distribution of finances under different laws and insurance options are a confusing maze and parents are often left alone to seek different types of financial support.

Case management is a huge task for social workers because of the nature of service delivery for these families. Families with children with severe disabilities may have to juggle ten to twenty different specialists for services in addition to the developmental and educational needs of their children. Service coordination is a major need for these families. Equally important are early intervention, initiating of support groups, transition planning, and advocacy (Beckman, 1996; Biggs, 1997; Lynn, 1994; Thyer and Kropf, 1995; Trivette et al., 1995).

Early intervention services are mandated by law and delivered in a team approach. Social work practitioners work as service coordinators within these teams. Initiation of support groups helps families relate to other with similar experiences. Transition planning is important once the child moves from a school setting to work and explores possibilities of independent living. Advocacy is necessary in all life stages of these families.

Orgassa (2001) found that families have a high need for such services provided by social workers as provision of sibling services and child care, sensitivity training for and education of the community, brokering, and crisis intervention.

Sibling services are necessary because siblings need to come to terms with the previously identified issues concerning their brother or sister with the disability. In addition to this, they have to discover who they are and establish a meaningful place within the family system. Also, siblings face the common problems and pressures that other children and adolescents face. Attention needs to be paid to those concerns as well. Related to sibling services is the issue of child care. Child care is necessary for both the children with disabilities and their siblings.

Sensitivity training for and education of the community can make living within this larger system easier for the families with children with disabilities. A community that is knowledgeable about disabilities and the rights of the persons with disabilities may be less likely to engage in stereotypes and alienation.

Brokering is especially helpful to families who have little or no experience with the service system, and who are overwhelmed by the availability or nonavailability of services, different eligibility criteria, and time lines. Social workers can use brokering together with service coordination as a major support for families navigating the complicated system of service provision.

Crisis intervention is a service that must be used as the last line of defense. It needs to be fast and thorough and will most likely lead to continuing treatment to alleviate the causes of the acute crisis situation. The causes do not necessarily have to lead back to the child with the disability. Other causes that social workers are familiar with can also be addressed, such as marriage problems, substance abuse problems, or mental illness.

Orgassa (2001) also identified qualities regarding service provision that families want in social workers. Most of these qualities are in accordance with the family-centered principles established earlier in the chapter. Some can also be considered common rules of conduct. The identified qualities were

- being on time for the interview or visit;
- focusing on the concern the family brought in;
- listening to the family;
- being sensitive to the issues the family raises;
- taking the family seriously;
- including the whole family;
- being positive and encouraging in their responses;
- going the "extra mile";
- learning and trying to understand the specific situation;

- being appreciative of the stresses the family is under;
- doing follow up on what was talked about;
- being creative in problem solving;
- being comfortable with the child; and
- being helpful (p. 172).

Social workers who adhere to these qualities will be very likely to find cooperative families in their practice. The families in the study attested that the majority of social workers they met had at least some of these qualities.

Even though the way in which services are provided makes a very big difference, it is also important that social workers know they are doing. Therefore, the study also looked at items the families thought social workers should have knowledge of or experience with. Those items were

- the disability of the child;
- the developmental level of the child;
- how to communicate with the child;
- emotional issues like loss, grief, or depression;
- sensitive issues like anger;
- the way the family interacts;
- medical implications;
- financial resources;
- legal issues;
- services in the community; and
- other families with similar experiences (Orgassa, 2001, p. 173).

In this list families focused on both the social workers as immediate service providers and as resources to other support systems. This utilization of social workers by families has led to positive outcomes for the families. In this study (Orgassa, 2001) a comparison between families who had contact with social workers with families who did not showed that the families with social worker contact had a significantly higher access to other service providers as well.

Social workers who are knowledgeable about the specific issues and stressors that families with children with disabilities face, who operate under a systems perspective, and who understand family-centered service provision can and will make a positive difference in the lives of the families with children with disabilities.

REFERENCES

Affleck, G. and Tennen, H. (1993). Cognitive adaptation to adversity: Insights from parents of medically fragile infants. In Turnbull, A. P., Patterson, J. M., Behr, S. K., Murphy, D. L., Marquis, J. G., and Blue-Banning, M. J. (Eds.), *Cognitive coping, families, and disability* (pp. 135-150). Baltimore, MD: Paul H. Brookes.

Alexander, R. and Tomkins-McGill, P. (1987). Notes to the experts from the parent of a handicapped child. *Social Work, 32,* 361-362.

Antonovsky, A. (1993). The implications of salutogenesis: An outsider's view. In Turnbull, A. P., Patterson, J. M., Behr, S. K., Murphy, D. L., Marquis, J. G., and Blue-Banning, M. J. (Eds.), *Cognitive coping, families, and disability* (pp. 111-122). Baltimore, MD: Paul H. Brookes.

Beckman, P. J. (1996). *Strategies for working with families of young children with disabilities.* Baltimore, MD: Paul H. Brookes.

Biggs, M. H. (1997). Building early intervention teams: Working together for children and families. In Butler, K. G. (Ed.), *Excellence in practice series.* Gaithersburg, MD: Aspen.

Boss, P. (1993). Boundary ambiguity: A block to cognitive coping. In Turnbull, A. P., Patterson, J. M., Behr, S. K., Murphy, D. L., Marquis, J. G., and Blue-Banning, M. J. (Eds.), *Cognitive coping, families, and disability* (pp. 257-286). Baltimore, MD: Paul H. Brookes.

Bristol, M. M., Gallagher, J. J., and Schopler, E. (1988). Mothers and fathers of young developmentally disabled and nondisabled boys: Adaptation and spousal support. *Developmental Psychology, 24,* 441-451.

Brown, J. D. (1993). Coping with stress: The beneficial role of positive illusions. In Turnbull, A. P., Patterson, J. M., Behr, S. K., Murphy, D. L., Marquis, J. G., and Blue-Banning, M. J. (Eds.), *Cognitive coping, families, and disability* (pp. 123-134). Baltimore, MD: Paul H. Brookes.

Corrigan, D. and Bishop, K. K. (1997). Creating family-centered integrated service systems and interprofessional educational programs to implement them. *Social Work in Education, 19,* 149-161.

Cowan, C. P. and Cowan, P. A. (2000). *When partners become parents: The big life changes for couples.* Mahwah, NJ: Lawrence Erlbaum Associates, Publishers.

Dempsey, I. (1996). Facilitating empowerment in families with a member with a disability. *Developmental Disabilities Bulletin, 24,* 1-19.

Dunst, C. J., Trivette, C. M., and Deal, A. G. (1994). *Supporting and strengthening families.* Volume 1: *Methods, strategies and practices.* Cambridge, MA: Brookline Books.

Dunst, C. J., Trivette, C. M., Hamby, D., and Pollock, B. (1990). Family-systems correlates of the behavior of young children with handicaps. *Journal of Early Intervention, 14,* 204-218.

Dunst, C. J., Trivette, C. M., Starnes, A. L., Hamby, D. W., and Gordon, N. J. (1993). *Building and evaluating family support initiatives: A national study of programs for persons with developmental disabilities.* Baltimore, MD: Paul H. Brookes.

Dunst, C. J., Trivette, C. M., and Thompson, R. L. (1990). Supporting and strengthening family functioning: Toward a congruence between principles and practice. *Prevention in Human Services, 9,* 19-43.

Ell, K. (1984). Social networks, social support, and health status: A review. *Social Service Review, 58,* 133-149.

Glasberg, B. A. and Harris, S. L. (1997). Grandparents and parents assess the development of their child with autism. *Child and Family Behavior Therapy, 19,* 17-27.

Herman, S. E. and Marcenko, M. O. (1997). Perceptions of services and resources as mediators of depression among parents of children with developmental disabilities. *Mental Retardation, 35,* 458-467.

Herman, S. E. and Thompson, L. (1995). Families' perception of their resources for caring for children with developmental disabilities. *Mental Retardation, 33*(2), 73-83.

Hill, R. (1949). *Families under stress.* New York: Harper & Row.

Hill, R. (1958). Generic features of families under stress. *Social Casework, 49,* 139-150.

Honig, A. S. and Winger, C. J. (1997). A professional support program for families of handicapped preschoolers: Decrease in maternal stress. *The Journal of Primary Prevention, 17,* 285-296.

Johnson, B. H. (1990). The changing role of families in health care. *Children's Health Care, 19,* 234-241.

Kalyanpur, M. and Rao, S. S. (1991). Empowering low-income black families of handicapped children. *American Journal of Orthopsychiatry, 61,* 523-532.

Lazarus, R. S. and Folkman, S. (1984). *Stress, appraisal and coping.* New York: Springer.

Levy, J. M., Rimmerman, A., Botuck, S., Ardito, M., Freeman, S. E., and Levy, P. H. (1996). The support network of mothers of younger and adult children with mental retardation and developmental disabilities receiving case management. *The British Journal of Developmental Disabilities, 82,* 24-31.

Leyser, Y. (1994). Stress and adaptation in orthodox Jewish families with a disabled child. *American Journal of Orthopsychiatry, 64*(3), 376-385.

Lightburn, A. and Pine, B. A. (1996). Supporting and enhancing the adoption of children with developmental disabilities. *Children and Youth Services Review, 18*(1/2), 139-162.

Lynn, G. L. (1994) The parents group: Coping with the developmentally disabled adolescent. *Journal of Child and Adolescent Group Therapy, 4,* 147-156.

Marsh, D. T. (1992). *Families and mental retardation: New directions in professional practice.* New York: Praeger.

Mausner, S. (1995). Families helping families: An innovative approach to the provision of respite care for families of children with complex medical needs. *Social Work in Pediatrics, 21,* 95-106.

McBride, S. L., Brotherson, M. J., Joanning, H., Whiddon, D., and Demmitt, A. (1993). Implementation of family-centered services: Perceptions of families and professionals. *Journal of Early Intervention, 17*(4), 414-430.

McCallion, P. and Toseland, R. W. (1993). Empowering families of adolescents and adults with developmental disabilities. *Families in Society: The Journal of Contemporary Human Services, 74,* 579-587.

McCubbin, H. I. and Figley, C.R. (1983). Bridging normative and catastrophic stress. In McCubbin, H. I. and Figley, C. R. (Eds.), *Stress and the family: Coping with normative transitions* (pp. 218-228). New York: Brunner/Mazel.

McCubbin, H. I., and Patterson, J. M. (1983). Family transitions: Adaptation to stress. In McCubbin, H. I. and Figley, C. R. (Eds.), *Stress and the family: Coping with normative transitions* (pp. 5-25). New York: Brunner/Mazel.

McCubbin, H. I., Thompson, E. A., Thompson, A. I., and McCubbin, M. A. (1993). Family schema, paradigms, and paradigm shifts: Components and processes of appraisal in family adaptation crises. In Turnbull, A. P., Patterson, J. M., Behr, S. K., Murphy, D. L., Marquis, J. G., and Blue-Banning, M. J. (Eds.), *Cognitive coping, families, and disability* (pp. 239-256). Baltimore, MD: Paul H. Brookes.

Meyer, D. J. (1993). Lessons learned: Cognitive coping strategies of overlooked family members. In Turnbull, A. P., Patterson, J. M., Behr, S. K., Murphy, D. L., Marquis, J. G., and Blue-Banning, M. J. (Eds.), *Cognitive coping, families, and disability* (pp. 81-94) . Baltimore, MD: Paul H. Brookes.

Orgassa, U. C. (2001). Social services for families with children with developmental disabilities: What is the consumer perspective? (Doctoral Dissertation, The University of Alabama, 2001). *Dissertation Abstracts International, 62*(03A): p. 1212.

Pardeck, J. and Yuen, F. (1997). A family health approach to social work practice. *Family Therapy, 2*(24), 115-128.

Pardeck, J. and Yuen, F. (Eds.) (1999). *Family health: A holistic approach to social work practice.* Westport, CT: Auburn House.

Pardeck, J., Yuen, F., Daley, J., and Hawkins, C. (1998). Social work assessment and intervention through family health practice. *Family Therapy, 1*(25), 25-39.

Pargament, K. I. (1990). God help me: Toward a theoretical framework of coping for the psychology of religion. *Social Scientific Study of Religion, 2,* 195-224.

Patterson, J. M. (1993). The role of family meanings in adaptation to chronic illness and disability. In Turnbull, A. P., Patterson, J. M., Behr, S. K., Murphy, D. L., Marquis, J. G., and Blue-Banning, M. J. (Eds.), *Cognitive coping, families, and disability* (pp. 221-238). Baltimore, MD: Paul H. Brookes.

Pearlin, L. I. and Turner, H. A. (1987). The family as a context of the stress process. In Kasl, S.V. and Cooper, C. L. (Eds.), *Stress and health: Issues in research methodology* (pp. 143-165). New York: John Wiley & Sons.

Petr, C. G. (1994). Crises that threaten out-of-home placement of children with emotional and behavioral disorders. *Families in Society, 75,* 195-203.

Petr, C. G. (1998). *Social work with children and their families.* New York: Oxford University Press.

Schilmoeller, G. L. and Baranowski, M. D. (1998). Intergenerational support in families with disabilities: Grandparents' perspectives. *Families in Society, 79,* 465-476.

Schulz, J. B. (1993). Heroes in disguise. In Turnbull, A. P., Patterson, J. M., Behr, S. K., Murphy, D. L., Marquis, J. G., and Blue-Banning, M. J. (Eds.), *Cognitive coping, families, and disability* (pp. 31-42). Baltimore, MD: Paul H. Brookes.

Seligman, M. and Darling, R. B. (1997). *Ordinary families, special children: A systems approach to childhood disability,* Second edition. New York: Guilford Press.

Thyer, B. A. and Kropf, N. P. (Eds.) (1995). *Developmental disabilities: A handbook for interdisciplinary practice.* Cambridge, MA: Brookline Books.

Traustadottir, R. (1995). A mother's work is never done: Constructing a "normal" family life. In Taylor, S.J., Bogdan, R., and Lutfiyya, Z. M. (Eds.), *The variety of community experience: Qualitative studies of family and community life* (pp. 23-46). Baltimore, MD: Paul H. Brookes.

Trivette, C. M., Dunst, C. J., Boyd, K., and Hamby, D. W. (1995). Family-oriented program models, helpgiving practices, and parental control appraisals. *Exceptional Children, 62,* 237-248.

Turnbull, A. P., Patterson, J. M., Behr, S. K., Murphy, D. L., Marquis, J. G., and Blue-Banning, M. J. (Eds.) (1993). *Cognitive coping, families, and disability.* Baltimore, MD: Paul H. Brookes.

Vohs, J. (1993). On belonging: A place to stand, a gift to give. In Turnbull, A. P., Patterson, J. M., Behr, S. K., Murphy, D. L., Marquis, J. G., and Blue-Banning, M. J. (Eds.), *Cognitive coping, families, and disability* (pp. 51-66). Baltimore, MD: Paul H. Brookes.

Yuen, F., Skibinski, G., and Pardeck, J. (Eds.) (2003). *Family health social work practice: A knowledge and skills casebook.* Binghamton, NY: The Haworth Press.

Chapter 6

Understanding Children's Reactions to Loss: A Holistic Approach

Joyce Burris

INTRODUCTION

Loss is an inevitable part of the experience of being human. As humans we experience loss because we form attachments and because we develop satisfying expectations about our lives and our loved ones. When our expectations change, or our lives and loved ones change, we cling to expectations that no longer fit reality and we experience loss as a result. When attachments are severed or our expectations are dashed or never realized, the complex process of grieving sets in. Humans at every age have the capacity to experience loss and to grieve (Furman, 1974; Shapiro, 1994; Sullivan, 1972).

Bowlby (1961) studied children's grief reactions in England during World War II observing the responses of children separated from parents and sent to safety in the countryside during the bombing of London. Bowlby documented the problems that these separations caused the children. Signs of distress and depression were witnessed by Bowlby and later included in his concept of separation anxiety (1960). He even identified phases in the mourning process that are similar to those of present-day theories about grief in adults. The first phase put the children in shock and disbelief that the loss had occurred, and the children showed signs of emotional numbness. When the reality of the separation began to sink in, there was a realization of the actuality of the loss and children articulated the loss explicitly. At the same time, the children expressed longings and yearnings for reunion with the lost parents. This was followed by disorganization and depression. Eventually there was an adjustment phase that allowed the children to connect with others in the new environment even while still missing their parents.

Bowlby's work has had an impact on medical practitioners who previously separated and isolated sick or injured children during hospitalizations while severely limiting or denying family contact (Bowlby, 1980). Practitioners currently try to include parents and family in the treatment of children as much as possible, owing to the importance of attachment in the developmental process, but also because family support speeds medical recovery.

The grieving process in children is similar in many ways to that of adults, but it is different in other ways (Dyregrov, 1991; Hatter, 1996; Hurd, 1999; Sanders, 1995; Silverman, 2000; Worden, 1996; Worden and Silverman, 1996). Losses are not easy to understand and are hard to face at any age, but children may have more difficulties overcoming loss because they do not have well-developed experiences and coping skills to see them through. Children depend upon adults for care and guidance, but frequently adults, who may themselves not understand how children experience and process loss, cannot adequately help the child who is grieving. Therefore, the purpose of this chapter is to highlight ways to understand and help children deal with loss and grief.

Ordinarily, grief and grieving are conceptualized in the context of a variety of losses. However, the death of a loved one is more challenging for a young person to accept. Parental death is no doubt the most difficult death for a child to face, and if that death is sudden, it is even harder for a child to process (Worden, 1996). In one study, it is suggested that close to 5 percent of children in the United States experience the death of a parent before the age of eighteen (Silverman and Worden, 1992). In another study, it was estimated that as high as 20 percent of children experience the death of a parent before age eighteen (Goldman, 2000). Indeed, the death of a loved one, whether that person is a parent or other person to whom the child is attached, is very difficult for children to grieve. Other losses affect children's emotional, social, behavioral, cognitive, and spiritual lives, and the grief response follows all types of losses that children encounter. These losses, such as the loss or death of pets, moving away from friends and family, having a sibling go off to college, experiencing the loss of innocence upon discovering historical and present-day atrocities that have been committed, or leaving home for the first day of preschool are examples of the experiences children grieve. Acknowledging the variety of causes that trigger the grief response is important. However, in this chapter, most of the discussion about children's grief responses will focus on reactions to the dying process and death, as it is the most challenging.

As children learn about their reactions and find ways to understand the events of their lives, they construct meanings and coping skills that give them an experience base from which to face future challenges (Nickman, Silverman, and Normand, 1998; Normand, Silverman, and Nickman, 1996). Children do not construct meanings and coping skills by themselves. They live their lives within the context of families, neighborhoods, communities, cultural groupings, and societies that provide models for how to cope, measures for appropriate behavior, and philosophical and spiritual meanings that are presented as culturally advisable ways to feel, behave, and to understand loss (DeSpelder and Strickland, 2002; Klass, 1996; Neuberger, 1987; Rosenblatt, 1993; Rosenblatt, Walsh, and Jackson, 1976). Although it is beyond the scope of this chapter to provide detailed descriptions of different cultural views and rituals regarding mourning, a second purpose of this chapter is to recognize that culturally diverse contexts in which children learn rituals and specific ways of grieving are important to them and their community.

Children cope differently at different ages. Indeed, preverbal children are likely to show somatic symptoms of distress in response to separation from a loved one. Play behavior and emotional expressions are the primary form of communication for very young children. Signs of depression, unresponsiveness to new caregivers, and search behaviors are witnessed in infants who experienced losses (Silverman, 2000). Children's grief responses are varied, among other things, in terms of intensity and length of time experienced. Many factors influence differences in the grief response and may include the following:

1. the type of loss and rituals in cultural context;
2. the relationship of the child with the lost object or person;
3. the relative centrality of the lost object of person;
4. the family influences, including role distribution in the family, communication, styles of reacting with loss, other stressors, de-

gree of disruption to the family functioning the loss represents, family cohesion, size, etc.;
5. community context, including supportiveness for the family and child who are experiencing loss; and
6. the child's age, sex, self-awareness, coping skills, perceptions, etc. (Worden, 1996).

Therefore, a third purpose of this chapter is to explore the grief reactions of children at various ages so as to understand how the developmental process affects grief reactions in children.

CULTURAL PRACTICES
AND THE ROLE OF CHILDREN

In Western cultures in the nineteenth century, the practices and rituals of grieving were more likely to occur in public, to include the entire extended family and community, and were likely to take place over extended periods of time. This historical period was called the age of the "beautiful death," according to Aries (1981). Mourners wore dark clothing to mark the significance of a death to the community in which the mourner lived. Family visits to the gravesite were frequent and rituals of mourning were flowery. Children embroidered wall hangings to memorialize a family member who died and the entire family sat around the bed of the dying person, prepared the body for community members to pay respects, and did much of the funeral preparation themselves (DeSpelder and Strickland, 2002).

However, that openness changed in the twentieth century, and for some time in Western culture it has been a common practice to exclude children from open, direct discussion about loss and death. Although this practice appears to be changing again, some parents and family friends still try to "protect" children from the realities of death or loss by avoiding the subject, by not talking about the grandparent with the terminal illness, by using euphemisms to brush the subject aside, or by sending the child away during the illness and dying process of a family member (DeSpelder and Strickland, 2002; Silverman, 2000; Worden, 1996). Children who are excluded from discussions about losses are left to struggle with their fears and anxieties in .isolation as they try to find meaning for the avoidant or secretive behaviors of the adults around them. When emotions are expressed, validated, and discussed openly, there is relief that is usually followed by an eventual ability to move beyond the loss with increased capacity to cope.

In some cultures today, honoring the dead is carried out in public ceremonies that last several days every year. Examples include the yearly Mexican and Mexican American celebrations of *Dia de los Muertos,* or Day of the Dead, that is held from October 31 through November 2, and the Japanese late summer traditions of *O-bon* for which the community gathers together to remember those who have died and live on in memory and spirit as revered ancestors. Children as well as entire families are included in the rituals and preparations for these community festivities in both Mexican and Japanese traditions (DeSpelder and Strickland, 2002).

It is a Mexican tradition to decorate food and almost anything else with skeleton figures for the Day of the Dead, and during other daily life events skeletons are used as a reminder that at any person might die at any time. Since everyone dies in the end, death is viewed as the great equalizer between rich and poor, men and women, bosses and workers, and is treated with sarcastic humor. The Japanese traditions are a more serious recognition of the connection of the living family members with the dead ancestors whereby lamps are lit to guide the spirits on their journey home.

Although the United States contains numerous cultural groups and communities that generate a wide variety of attitudes, rituals, and practices about death and dying, the practice of the "hidden death" seems to prevail (DeSpelder and Strickland, 2002). Immigrants who come to the United States and want to practice traditional ways are sometimes prohibited by the power of the funeral industry and its influence over local zoning and public health laws (Mitford, 1963).

It was during the twentieth century's "medicalization and professionalization of death" that death became increasingly hidden from public view. Medical personnel have been and still are trained to view death as a failure of science and of their inadequate skills or medical expertise rather than a natural process (Marrone, 1997). In the majority of deaths, professionals, rather than the family and community, attend to the care of the dying person. Medical practices concerning the dying person are emphasized in a controlled hospital setting in which care focuses primarily only on the physical symptoms of diseases, not the whole person. After death, professionals carry out most of the funeral services, with the family and community playing spectator roles.

The obvious challenge to this standard is the modern hospice movement that began in England as the result of work by medical social worker Dr. Cicely Saunders, who practiced medical care that focused on comfort and pain management with open awareness that the person is dying (Ingles, 1980). Hospice is holistic in that all the needs of the dying person are considered, including emotional, existential and spiritual, physical, mental, social and cultural, family, etc. and it is often practiced in the home of the person dying. The purpose is to provide the least restrictive and most comfortable environment for the dying person that does not focus only on medical treatment, as the majority of hospital environments do.

In the United States, grief is often equated with a disease or illness (Furman, 1974; Silverman, 2000; Volkan, 1981). Persons experiencing grief reactions are referred to medical or psychiatric specialists, or grieving individuals are contained within bereavement groups led by clinicians. Workplace environments give very limited time (usually only a few days) off for bereavement. Indeed, the message given in almost every institutional setting, including mental health settings, is that grief reactions should cause little disruption in public life and that if grief is experienced over an extensive period of time (i.e., more than six months), then it is pathological. These attitudes are not helpful to the grieving person at any age (Silverman, 2000).

The rise of the ideology of individualism is another change in Western culture that has marginalized the importance of community rituals and community involvement in mourning. Modern psychology, with its emphasis on separation, individual identity, and individual coping skills, has become a discipline that usually claims the role of educating the public on death and dying (Meyer, 1988; Parsons, 1994; Silverman, 2000). Grieving is described as being experienced by an individual alone rather than within a community, in which the larger social context matters. The focus is placed on inner and outer restraint of the individual who is encouraged to get through the grieving process as quickly and efficiently as possible. Meyer (1988) contends that the ideology of individualism in Western culture has more to do with economic, cultural, and political systems than with the well-being of the individual, family, community, or the nation.

THE GRIEVING PROCESS

Many psychological theories of grief initially rely on the work of Freud (1961), who emphasized the importance of detaching one's thoughts and memories of the deceased and letting go (decathexis) of emotional attachments in order to free up emotional energy so that the individual might form new relationships. Silverman and Klass (1996) found that in Freud's writings about his personal life, he found complete detachment impossible. Nonetheless, this concept has, until recently, remained in the psychological literature as an unquestioned assumption (Gilligan, 1993; Miller, 1986; Silverman, 2000).

Although grief is the natural response to loss, thanatologists have studied grief and have developed various models to understand the process. Models of grief have, until recently, included a series of sequential linear stages for experiencing grief reactions that suggest a correct way of grieving (Gorer, 1967; Kavanaugh, 1972; Kübler-Ross, 1969). Though each model differs from the others, they include similar descriptions of such stages as the following: shock, bargaining and denial, disorganization, preoccupation with the deceased, expression of volatile emotions (anger, guilt, loneliness), awareness and acceptance, depression and despair, relief, and reorganization of sense of self. However, current thinking acknowledges that individuals grieve in diverse and messy ways that do not necessarily follow the neat, stage-based models proposed in the previous generation.

Stroebe and Schut (1999) proposed a framework for grieving that they call the Dual-Process Model of Loss. Using the Dual-Process Model of Loss, grief is experienced as a dynamic rather than linear process. This description of grief views the mourning person as oscillating between focusing on or confronting and avoiding cues that evoke the pain of the grief reactions. The grieving person, regardless of age or culture, uses coping strategies that are both loss and restoration oriented, and these two coping methods are often used simultaneously. The griever struggles with two contrary emotions: to hold on to the loved but lost object, and to let go and accept that the relationship has ended.

The loss stressor requires a loss-oriented coping strategy whereby the individual, family, and community deal with the changes, both internal and external, caused by the loss. This might include attempts to focus on the loss experience in terms of reflections about the significance of the loss. The restoration stressors require making adjustments to the secondary consequences of the loss. In addition to their own role activities, surviving adults must take on tasks and roles formerly carried out by the ill or deceased person. This increases the load carried under already stressed conditions. Ideally, community members help in this endeavor by offering help in tangible ways (bringing food, helping with child care, donating money, etc.) and in intangible ways by being available for emotional support. Community reactions to the loss may change friendship patterns, social status, and communication lifelines, and many families are left to their own devices in dealing with loss (Silverman, 2000). Children may also take on additional tasks and roles in the household and may find that the remaining parent is so stressed in the face of loss that there is even less time for them to get the special attention they need.

Although adults share these adaptive responses, the following behaviors are considered normal for the child who is grieving according to Black (1996): "1. changes in appetite or sleep patterns; 2. withdrawal; 3. difficulty concentrating; 4. regression to an earlier developmental stage; 5. increased dependency; 6. restlessness; and 7. anger, anxiety, sadness, and aggression" (p. 302). Every child does not necessarily experience all of these symptoms, as the grieving process varies according to a number of factors, such as individual's age, personality, experience, and holistic developmental states; the nature of the loss; relationship of the bereaved with the person who died; social context; and community and family culture and support.

Worden (1996) identified four "tasks of mourning" that involve the abilities of the person in interaction with others to cope with loss. They include the following:

- Accepting the reality of the loss
- Working through the pain of grief
- Adjusting to a changed environment in which the deceased is missing
- Emotionally relocating the deceased and moving on with life (pp. 10-18)

WHAT HELPS TO SUPPORT CHILDREN
AS THEY GRIEVE?

Supporting children's efforts in grieving a loss strengthens bonds and allows children to know that they are not alone. What children need most to assist them as they move through the grieving process is someone to listen actively and permissively to them. Very young children communicate mostly on a nonverbal level, so it is important to not miss opportunities to see what their drawings and actions in play may be communicating. Children are generally very adept at perceiving inconsistencies between levels of communication. If they receive inconsistent messages they are more likely to internalize the nonverbal cues. Thus an important thing to do for children as they grieve is to be a good role model for how to talk about feelings, to communicate that grief is an appropriate response to loss, and to provide behaviors that allow the integration of grief reactions.

It does not help children to be told how to feel, think, or act. However, encouraging children to talk about their feelings, accepting them with positive regard, and being responsive to wherever they are in the grieving process can be very helpful. It is important to not overprotect children from loss, as most efforts to do so are likely to increase anxiety, fear, and confusion. Furthermore, loss is an inevitable aspect of life, and learning to adequately meet life's challenges will prepare children for the future. Children should be allowed information appropriate to their developmental level, out of which they may make choices about how to participate in mourning rituals. Forcing them to participate or to confront death beyond their abilities to integrate the experience may be traumatizing. Granted, traumatic events do happen to children despite efforts to create healthy protective environments for them, so being available to listen and to encourage young people to process their experiences is most helpful.

The concerns that children express are at root reflective of anxieties about surviving separation from nurturing adults (Bowlby, 1960). Children and teens need reassurance in both word and deed that they are not alone, and that in spite of loss, they are valued and loved.

At young ages (before ages six to eight) children think that they cause or are responsible for things that happen in their lives. It is important to address these beliefs directly and to let children know that just because they were mad at Grandpa and secretly wished for his death, that angry and expressed fleeting wishes do not cause death. Other reassurances may need to be given that there is no "right" way to grieve nor any recipe that they can follow that will quickly resolve the pain. Being available and responsive throughout the confusion of grief reactions and expressing concern and affection for the duration of the grieving process may be the most helpful gift a young person can receive.

Another helpful suggestion is to maintain as much as possible a normal routine of activities while allowing for more time to process the loss. Bedtime, mealtime, and other daily rituals give children a feeling of safety. These ritualized markers of normalcy help children regain their equilibrium and assist in restoring confidence that, in spite of loss, life does go on. Normal activities also provide temporary respite from the pain and stress of grieving. On the other hand, too much distraction from grief reactions, or attempts at replacing the loved lost person too quickly, will not allow time and space to do the important grief work that needs to be accomplished for children to integrate their loss. Excessive distractions would also send the message to a child that grieving should not be outwardly expressed. This sends the child underground to grieve in isolation or to cut off feelings prematurely.

Worden (1996) suggests that during the grieving process children need the following:

- adequate information,
- having their fears and anxieties addressed,
- careful listening,
- validation of individuals' feelings,
- help with overwhelming feelings,
- involvement and inclusion,
- continued routine activities,
- modeled grief behaviors, and
- opportunities to remember the deceased. (p. 91)

This list contains items that adults also need in the grieving process, which harkens back to the important point that children and adults grieve in some similar ways. The following section will address differences in the developmental process that highlight special needs that children have at various developmental periods.

GRIEVING CHILDREN
AND DEVELOPMENTAL ISSUES

Children experience the world in different ways at various points along the developmental life span and, thus, adults need to tailor their support for a grieving child based on the child's developmental processes (Attig, 1996). As previously stated, there is much variety in the ways that children grieve, with differences depending on family, cultural, and community modeling and support, and the child's personality, experience, and maturity, among other things. In tracing the changing attitudes and responses to loss and death in childhood, as well as the ways children may be supported at various developmental points along the way, it is useful to have theoretical perspectives on child development within which to discuss children's views. The two frameworks chosen for this discussion are symbolic interactionism and Piaget's theory on cognitive development.

Symbolic Interactionism

Symbolic interactionism is a theoretical perspective from sociology that has been used to understand how human beings develop. An assumption from this perspective is that humans are social beings and require social interaction for development and optimal well-being. Humans create symbols to further social interaction and then, out of shared experiences, imbue these created symbols with meaning. The importance of the social aspects of one's life, such as historical and social context, social space, and shared meanings, are observed by symbolic interactionists who emphasize the norms, social roles, cultural values, and beliefs that provide meaning to the developmental process of individuals.

Charles Horton Cooley (1909[1962]) developed a way of understanding children's sense of a "self" that he called "the looking glass self," as it is based on a reciprocal process of interaction between the individual and others who serve as representatives of society. The individual interprets symbolic feedback from others to get a sense of who they are as social "selves." Out of the information that is put together by the individual about the feedback they interpret from others, the individual chooses to act in ways that either agree with or contradict the social reflection they subjectively observe in the looking glass.

This theory is somewhat similar to the "self-fulfilling prophecy" used in psychology except, in symbolic interactionism, the individual is viewed as having a choice in the matter. The nature of the feedback is viewed as social, symbolic, and societal in Cooley's theory. In other words, a person born in another society, neighborhood, or historical period, with different cultural symbols and different shared meanings, would likely develop differently as the feedback to the individual comes out of shared meanings that are fundamentally social rather than merely psychological.

George Herbert Mead (1934) observed that child development took place in three phases: (1) imitation phase (birth to two years), (2) play phase (two to four years), and (3) game phase (four to six or seven years). During the imitation phase, babies imitate the shared gestures and behaviors that they see around them and that they experience in face-to face interaction. In the play phase, children start organizing the meanings of behaviors, social statuses, and roles into categories, so that when, for example, they play "fireman," they know which walk, tone of voice, gesture, behaviors, clothes, and other objects to use in order to act out the role of fireman. Children distinguish the symbols for fireman from those needed to act out other roles in society. In the game phase, children take the role of the "generalized other" or the internalized social audience to critique how well they are playing various roles. In other words, they step outside the role they are playing to reflect the evaluative attitudes of their social community. They critique how well they are playing the chosen role.

Symbolic interactionism provides an understanding of the importance of social relationships and the significance of community in helping individuals create a sense of self. Through social relationships, individuals learn to organize, validate, and define feelings, actions, values, and priorities for their lives. When a person experiences a loss, the person's very sense of self is at stake (Rosenblatt, 1993). A young child is vulnerable because he or she has not internalized a solid sense of self for lack of a large experiential palate called living. Children also need some direction to know how to make sense of a loss.

Helping children make choices about how to be involved in rituals of mourning allows children to participate in creating shared meaning. Children should know ahead of time what to expect before attending a memorial or funeral service. The symbolic meanings of such occasions can be confusing and overwhelming for children. Reassurance that the child will continue to be valued and loved is always helpful to children when delivered with sincerity. An understanding that the reciprocal creation of symbols is not only important to give meaning to the loss, but also to give meaning to the developing sense of self, can encourage participation of children in the process of experiencing a loss.

Piaget's Cognitive Developmental Theory

The work of Swiss psychologist Jean Piaget (1954) focused on the cognitive development of children and has had a profound effect on understanding children—particularly on understanding how children think things through at various ages. Piaget was an astute observer of children's problem-solving processes, observing them in their natural environments and carefully documenting his observations. His interest was not whether children solved a problem in a certain way or got a right answer according to some expert on a question; Piaget was most interested in how children work through to an answer for themselves.

Piaget conceptualized the basic building blocks of cognition as starting with what he called a *schema*. A schema functions similar to a computer file for organizing information into a meaningful structure. When a child encounters any new information, particularly information that challenges an existing schema, the individual is required to rethink the prior organization system to *accommodate* the new information. When the new understanding is firmly in place, the child is said to have *assimilated* the new information into a now altered and more elaborate schema. The process cycles and begins again when additional new information challenges the structure of understanding that the child has achieved. Thus, cognitive development involves a dynamic and active movement, or *cognitive transformation* that requires the individual to engage in constant processing, reconsidering, and reorganizing of information into an organizational structure that allows the child ready reference and requires constant reconceptualization.

Piaget conceptualized the developmental process as being one of *sequential stages of development or transformations* of the individual's worldview from birth to adolescence. Although the stages represent to Piaget fairly predictable changes that children go through in the developmental process, there is a great deal of diversity among children at the same age in their achievement of developmental skills to comprehend their world. Piaget did not hold hard and fast to the ages that coincide with the particular stages. He was more interested in the progression of cognitive skills involved in development than in calculating precise ages of achievement of particular levels. Piaget (1954) conceptualized the four stages of development or transformation as the following: (1) sensorimotor stage, (2) preoperational stage, (3) concrete operational stage, and (4) formal operations. Each stage represents the mastery of particular concepts:

1. *Sensorimotor* (birth to two years old): Child's abilities are primarily in the here and now. Child uses senses to take in information and relies on motor abilities to experiment in discovering how things work. In the first month the child is limited to reflexive actions (sucking, crying, sneezing), but with abilities to walk, run, climb, pick things up, and with beginning language skills, by eighteen to twenty-four months can create *mental representations* and starts using the imagination to problem solve. Somewhere close to midway develops *object permanence,* which is the understanding that even when objects are not seen, they continue to exist. Child uses trial and error at this stage to figure things out, and by twelve months is actively engaged in solving new problems.

2. *Preoperational* (two to seven years old): *Centration* occurs at this stage, during which a child tends to see only one aspect of an object at a time. This shows up in *classification skills*. The child cannot comprehend that his mother can also be someone's daughter and someone's sister at the same time.
   - *Egocentrism* is the quality of thinking whereby a child focuses on his or her own direct experience and is not able to think from the point of view of someone else. If child has not experienced something he or she has difficulty hypothetically thinking about it.
   - *Symbolic functioning* refers to a child's ability to use language to understand his or her surroundings, and to use one

object to represent another (e.g., a wooden block becomes a car). The child is rather literal in the way he or she understands language and applies meaning to situations.

- *Deferred imitation* refers to a child's ability to store a mental image of something and then to imitate it much later. (e.g., a child watches another feed the goat at a petting zoo and a week later imitates the feeding behavior with the goat).
- *Irreversability* suggests that a child at this stage cannot reverse logic easily to apply it to the reverse case.
- *Conservation of matter:* The child cannot understand that by changing the shape of something that its volume is not affected.

3. *Concrete operations* (seven to twelve years old):
   - *Conservation of matter:* The child understands that the shape or container holding something does not affect the amount or quantity of that substance.
   - *Classification skills:* The child is more able to handle many aspects or qualities of something at one time and is more able to reflect others' points of view.
   - *Concrete thinking:* The child interprets facts concretely and literally but still cannot understand the gray areas of life very well, and cannot think abstractly very well.

4. *Formal operations* (teen years): The child can think *hypothetically, abstractly,* and *logically,* and can pick out logical inconsistencies. The child at this stage uses both deductive and inductive reasoning and can plan ahead and think through to logical consequences. The child is more able to understand many points of view at the same time (relativistic thinking) and can handle multiple steps at multiple levels necessary for higher-level math.

Infancy and Toddler Years

The first two years of life are generally dominated by sensations that are experienced through the baby's body. The infant cannot yet utilize language to understand or describe to others what is happening. However, babies do put together meaning for themselves, and when there is a disruption of their routine or a person to whom they are attached is absent, they show their displeasure by crying, being restless, or by any number of other responses. As the child's motor abilities develop, learning becomes much more active. A child can grab a stick, and shaking it at one end, be surprised that the other end moves. Observing this the child learns something about cause and effect. The child also learns to see the ways in which she or he has an impact on the surrounding environment. Although language limitations exist and children cannot communicate verbally to others what they know or understand, infants can communicate nonverbally.

Children at this age show their response to loss through bodily symptoms and somatic complaints that are similar to those suffered by bereaved adults. These responses might include lack of appetite, insomnia, nausea, restlessness, general crankiness, emotional withdrawal, crying, and regression to earlier outgrown behaviors. Children who suffer loss of caregivers or have inadequate caregivers who do not bond with them may exhibit what is called "failure to thrive." Children who do not experience a close intimate relationship with a caregiver will not have their survival needs met (food, water, shelter, warmth, personal hygiene), and they will not gain weight or grow normally. They waste away and can ultimately die. In the meantime, they withdraw, stare off in space, and become depressed. Bonding is crucial for survival and development.

It is possible to reverse this neglectful situation by providing a close and loving relationship with the infant in which bonding can take place. Some children are resilient and some caregivers are very effective at establishing the bonds necessary to restore the child. For less traumatic losses, the comfort of physical touch and a calm voice (either speaking softly, reading, or singing) can be helpful. Infants experience reassurance through touch. Baby massage is a good way to communicate a sense of connectedness and well-being to help a baby deal with a loss. Routines give infants a feeling of safety, so establishing routines is always a good idea.

Early Childhood

This is the *preoperational stage* according to Piaget (1954), when the child's realities are egocentric or only understood from his or her own direct experiences. It is not uncommon for children at this age to think that they did something to cause life events to happen. They take things literally at this age. Adults are surprised at the number of phrases or clichés used in everyday chatter that refer to death and are misunderstood by children. Consider the following example of a very young child who is coming to understand death (Brent, 1977). Luckily, the boy's father is very skilled in how he handles the situation.

A young boy has been waking up several times every night for a couple of months, asking for a bottle of sugar water after engaging in screaming behavior. The father was perplexed, as the child had previously been sleeping through the night for some many months. He lifted the child out of the crib, held him comfortably, and probed the child as to why this might be happening. After some coaxing, the child said he wanted the water so he could "make contact." The father was confused and asked what "make contact" meant. The child said, "If I run out of gas, I can't make contact—my engine won't go. You know!" The father still did not understand and asked the boy why he was afraid that he would run out of gas. To which the boy replied that he was afraid if he did not have gas, his motor will die.

Finally the father remembered that some time before he was selling an old car to a possible buyer who could not get the motor to turn over. In the presence of his son, he had advised the buyer to give it more juice, but as it turned out, the battery was "dead" because it wouldn't "make contact." The father, realizing that the boy had taken these phrases literally, hugged the boy, and asked him directly if he was afraid that he would die if he did not get juice. The boy was still crying when he said that he was indeed afraid that he would die if he ran out of gas.

The father then explained that people are different than cars, and that people can run two and maybe three days without eating and not die. He then explained that cars have keys that can be used to turn off motors and asked the boy, "Where is the key to turn you on and off?" Recognizing that he had none, the father explained to the boy that, unlike a car, he didn't need a key, and teased him that his belly button would be a good place for a key. The father and the son laughed. The father asked the boy if he could be turned off and on, and discovering that the son was not like a car, gave his son permission to sleep. The son went to sleep with no further screaming in the middle of that or any other night. Just for good measure, the father predicted that his son's motor would still be running in the morning and that he could sleep without worrying.

As it turns out, this father had earlier used the metaphor of a motor dying to explain to the boy why his pet parakeet died. Thus, the boy had witnessed death as a very powerful experience in direct connection with hearing the metaphor.

This leads into another piece of advice in dealing with death or loss with children. It is not a good idea to take away a child's fantasies or to create fantasies about loss or death. It is better to work with the child's images so as to clarify confusions. Asking children questions about the fantasy they may have created helps them to question any discrepancies they may not have seen, and makes it more likely that they will express deeper levels of understanding. Children may temporarily need the fantasy they have created until they get to a deeper level of understanding and acceptance.

There is the risk that an adult, in creating fantasies about loss for a child, may create a situation in which, instead of being comforted, the child may take the fantasy literally, misunderstand, and as a result become more fearful, anxious, guilt ridden, or confused. It is always good to keep listening, talking, and probing children to clear up misunderstandings. The father in the previous example kept asking questions because he knew there had to be some great disturbance in his son's mind for him to be waking every night. He listened carefully and looked for the hidden meanings in his son's explanations of what was happening.

Drawing pictures or creating an art project can help children express their feelings. Always let children talk about their creations, and in that conversation unresolved feelings will likely emerge. Be aware that children's feelings may come out in their drawings and paintings, but do not overinterpret. Let them tell you what they mean.

Body mutilation is a common fear for children at the preoperational age since they are just gaining mastery over their own body functions. This is important for their self-image. The child at this age is seeking answers for why things happen and how things work, and they are very interested to find their place in the explanations.

In order to understand how Piaget's concepts apply to this stage of development, Koocher (1973) (as reported in DeSpelder and Strickland, 2002) asked children at various ages to answer the question, "What makes things die?" From the following answers the reader observes the struggles that children engage in to understand abstract ideas about death. Their answers show how incompletely children understand death, but at the same time reveal ways adults might interact with children regarding these subjects.

Children at Piaget's preoperational stage responded to the question "What makes things die?" by giving the following answers:

NANCY: When they eat bad things, like if you went with a stranger and they gave you a candy bar with poison on it.
RESEARCHER: Anything else?
NANCY: Yes, you can die if you swallow a dirty bug.

CAROL: They eat poison and stuff, pills. You'd better wait until your Mom gives them to you.

RESEARCHER: Anything else?

CAROL: Drinking poison water and stuff like going swimming alone.

DAVID: A bird might get real sick and die if you catch it.

RESEARCHER: Anything else?

DAVID: They could eat the wrong foods like aluminum foil. That's all I can think of. (DeSpelder and Strickland, 2002, p. 351)

These answers are indicative of the egocentrism of the preoperational stage, and they also contain the characteristics of magical thinking and fantasy reasoning. One can certainly decipher the messages of caution these children have received from caregivers, and not minding authority certainly seems to be fraught with hazard in these children's minds. Children think that when bad things happen, they caused them. Symbolic interactionists would also point out that in the United States a well-known cultural message is given that Santa knows "who has been bad or good" and only brings toys to good boys and girls.

Death is somewhat tied into fantasies of reversibility. In fact, most researchers do not think that children think of death as permanent until around the age of seven. This is also the age at which children understand the concept of conservation of matter. Conservation of matter allows children to understand permanency of materials.

Middle Childhood Years

In Piaget's model, children from ages seven to twelve years are in the *concrete operational stage.* This is the stage at which children begin to use logic, however shakily, to solve problems. Children are still somewhat egocentric and tend to understand only what they have directly experienced. However, they are aware that others have experiences that may differ from their own. They better understand time and can remember the past and predict into the future. Their classification skills are improving. They are still not able to think hypothetically or abstractly to a great degree. The tendency to classify things in either/or terms is a characteristic that is typical of this stage.

In Koocher's (1973) study (as reported in DeSpelder and Strickland, 2002, p. 352) children answered the question, "What makes things die?" with the following:

TODD: Knife, arrow, guns, and lots of stuff. You want me to tell you all of them?

RESEARCHER: As many as you want.

TODD: Hatchets, and animals, and fires and explosions, too.

KENNY: Cancer, heart attacks, poison, guns, bullets, or if someone drops a boulder on you.

DEBORAH: Accidents, cars, guns, or a knife. Old age, sickness, taking dope, or drowning.

At this stage, death becomes more factual and realistic and the answers are delivered in a matter-of-fact way (Silverman, 2000). However, the unmistakable impact of the special effects shown in movies and cartoons is also present in these answers. Death is seen as permanent and universal. However, there are still feelings of guilt at this stage in thinking that they may have caused a death by wishing for someone's death in an angry moment. They have developed principles of what is "right" and "wrong" and view death as punishment for bad behavior. Reactions vary from being critical to sensitive, silly to morbid. Awareness is growing that death cannot be wished away magically.

Adolescence

In Piaget's model, *formal operations* represents the maturation of the cognitive process. Abstract thought, hypothetical thinking, logical problem solving, ability to plan in the future, and ability to carry out manipulations of ideas on many levels adds up to maturity according to Piaget. Teens can now understand another's point of view in the real world and can see that relationships go through ups and downs. Teens are more independent in their thought and can easily spot logical inconsistencies. To the question that Koocher posed, "What makes things die?" (as reported in DeSpelder and Strickland, 2002, p. 353) teens answered with the following:

ED: You mean death in a physical sense?

RESEARCHER: Yes.

ED: Destruction of a vital organ or life force within us.

GEORGE: They get old and their body gets all worn out, and their organs don't work as well as they used to.

PAULA: When the heart stops, blood stops circulating. You stop breathing, and that's it.

RESEARCHER: Anything else?

PAULA: Well there's lots of ways it can get started, but that's what really happens.

Teens have a more factual understanding of death. However, one of the struggles for teens is to know where they belong in the world and who they want to "be" as adults. Their preoccupation is with the future, so a death or major loss is a big blow to their established concerns and thought processes. Also, limited life experience makes coping with death of a loved one emotionally difficult. At any of the stages of childhood and adolescence, books can be used as an aid to coping. Support groups are also helpful, particularly in the teen years, though community support is helpful at any age. There are also national organizations that can help children, families, and communities cope with losses of various kinds.

CONCLUSION

This chapter ends as it began, with the observation that loss and death are inevitable in the process of living. We cannot protect children from loss and from knowing about death. What we can do is plan for the necessary discussions about death and improve our knowledge so that we can be supportive in a helpful way. We can hone our listening skills and be present in the lives of children. We can create ways to reach out to young people in our community and develop visible symbols of caring so that young people will be encouraged to ask for help when needed. Counseling staff and social workers in schools can successfully reach out to young people. Programs that sponsor support groups for bereavement in community sites such as schools, hospitals, and churches can be helpful. Parent support groups in the community can help educate parents and help them better understand and support their children.

In 2004, presidential candidate and Ohio Representative Dennis Kucinich proposed the development of a Department of Peace. This department would be established to create a visible symbol that peace is important to our national identity, but it would also create practical policies and programs to address the underlying pain in families, in people's individual lives, and in the communities in which people live. Unacknowledged loss is most often what lies at the heart of pain. Too many individuals are motivated to think that violence is the only available response to pain. National and state child welfare policies have been established to protect children after violence, abuse, or neglect have occurred in the family, but we have little to prevent the violence from occurring. Few entities are available to help people understand the links among loss, pain, and violence that would help them achieve a more peaceful existence. Our current responses of providing shelters and foster homes constitute the institutionalization of too little, too late. A Department of Peace could potentially be a way to make these concerns more visible and more of a priority.

Richard Titmuss (1968), a British policy planner, defines policy as the integration of all efforts (individual, group, or collective) to achieve some valued goal that serves the public good. Policy, in other words, is what we do, not what we say we do in some bill or piece of legislation that grows dusty on a shelf. We need more collective interventions that serve the wider interests of society on this issue. To this end, the hospice movement is thriving, and television journalist Bill Moyers created a four-part national public broadcasting series on how to deal with, understand, and talk about death, illness, and loss within the family and community aimed specifically at health care providers. More needs to be done, and our creative efforts need to be applied to helping one another.

Case Example: The Death of a Parent

The death of a parent is difficult for an adult child to grieve, but for a very young child it is doubly hard to understand and accept. The death of a parent turns the family into a confusing place. The surviving parent is also grieving, is overwhelmed with making final arrangements, must deal with grieving children in the family, and at the same time is taking the first steps into single parenthood. There is great potential to create a situation in which a young child feels isolated and unsupported. A remaining parent who is established in a home that is owned and has a job that will continue to provide adequately for the family faces a very different reality than a parent who is losing a home due to the financial hardship of lost income or who has to look for or begin a new job. The double workload entailed in taking on the responsibilities of the deceased parent will inevitability create stress for the remaining parent, and will affect all family members.

As was discussed earlier, children grieve based on their own style, coping skills, personality, developmental status, and social context. In addition, they are influenced by the styles of grieving modeled by surviving family members, peers, and community members. How the remaining parent tells the child about the death depends on many factors including the degree of openness in communication within the family, whether or not an extended period of illness occurred before the death that would allow for preparatory grief to take place, community support available to the family, ability of the remaining parent to respond to the child's needs, family resources available, and the extent of the new responsibilities for the remaining parent.

Anticipating the Death

Jim, age nine, had long talks with his dad before his dad died of cancer. His father had utilized the services of hospice and had died at home where Jim could witness the six-month decline. Members of the hospice team also talked with Jim about preparing for his father's death and answered any questions that Jim had. This had been very helpful because Jim's mother was looking for a new job that would bring in the increased salary necessary for the family to keep their home.

News of the Death

When Jim's father died, Jim and his mother were sitting close by. Jim saw his father take his last breath while he and his mother were holding his father's hands. Now it was just the two of them. Jim needed some time to accept the reality of death. Even though he intellectually knew what to expect, he was shocked that his father was actually dead. He could not reconcile the lifelessness of his father's body with the acute memories of his playful and strong earlier self. Jim went into the backyard by himself, partly to hide his emotions but also to sort them out. As he sat on the swing that his father had built for him, he tried to understand his father's death.

Though it was difficult, his mother understood that Jim needed some time apart. It was difficult for her to be patient and concerned for Jim as a first priority when she was feeling so raw and fragile herself in dealing with the loss of a husband that she had been married to for more than fifteen years. However, she knew that for Jim to lose a father at such a young age would be hard on him also. Luckily, he had two uncles, a neighbor, two sets of grandparents, and lots of friends to help him. His teacher, Mr. Bolt, was also a wonderful person who had been very supportive. Jim's mother knew that she was not alone. The outpouring of love and support from the community was comforting even if it did not diminish her sorrow.

Accepting the Finality of Death

At Jim's age the knowledge that death is final is within his cognitive capacity. However, he struggles with the emotional acceptance of that reality. There are times when he wants to tell his dad something and runs into the room before remembering that his dad is never going to come back. He had dreams that seem very real and his dad is in them as he used to be in Jim's life. This makes Jim very sad. He cannot stop the memories from flooding into his awareness, taking him by surprise and causing him to cry. This is embarrassing when it happens at school with all his friends around, so he avoids his friends quite a bit. This makes him feel even more alone. What helps him is that his mother spends time with him every day when she gets home from work to let him talk, or to read to him, or go for a bike ride with him. On Sundays, they go to the lake where they sprinkled his father's ashes after the memorial service.

Connecting with His Father's Death and Memorializing His Father's Memory

Jim felt good when he decorated the inside of the wooden container that his dad was cremated in and drew pictures of all the things he used to share with his dad. This had been his mom's idea to include him in the last rites so Jim could be involved, say goodbye, and have one last chance to give his dad something of himself.

Maintaining Daily Routines

Jim's mother called on friends and family to help her with yard work, meals, home repairs, etc., so that she would have time for Jim. This was hard for her because she was so preoccupied with her own grief. She worried about whether she would be adequately responsive to Jim's needs. She did not want to burden Jim with her grief, yet she did not want to hide it from him. She joined a bereavement group to get the support she needed. The group made it easier for her to talk appropriately with Jim about her grief and still allow her to be receptive for him to address his grief. Her brothers took Jim to baseball games, to movies, out for pizza, and on overnights at their houses to give Jim a sense of a normal routine. This gave Jim's mom some time alone to deal with her own grief, and she really needed that. She tried as much as she could to maintain a consistent schedule of household and community activities to help Jim make the transition that he was working to make in accepting the loss of his dad and in restructuring a sense of self. She was doing the same for herself. She also tried to build in time for fun activities, knowing that there were times that she would have to cancel plans at the last minute because Jim would not be up to them. She did not push him. She was just available to him as much as she could be.

Transition to a New Sense of Self

While they were grieving, Jim and his mother felt like it would never end. Jim would feel the saddest when he would see the oak tree in the backyard that his dad had planted. He would also feel sad when he saw oak trees in the fields as he and his mother drove around town. His father loved nature and Jim remembered how his father protected trees when Jim was a small boy. Jim had wanted to build a tree house and had gathered supplies with his friends to do just that. His dad had told him that the living part of the tree was just under the bark and that a nail driven into the tree would be like puncturing his own skin. Jim remembered being frustrated by his dad's feelings about the tree at that time, but now that memory brings him in touch with his loss.

When people grieve, they poignantly feel that they have been cheated, that their relationship with the loved one has been cut short, and they cannot imagine ever feeling differently. If the survivors do not run away from facing their feelings, the transformation begins. Gradually, they are able to feel more of their own lives, imagine future hopes and dreams, and shift to feeling gratitude that they had the opportunity to have the beloved but lost person in their lives. That is an indication that the grieving process is coming to completion. Such a loss will affect the entire life of a person, especially one so young as nine years old losing someone as significant as a father, but it will gradually become part of the individual's life rather than the focal point.

Jim's dad had been dead for a year and an informal anniversary service had been held by his mom with the help of friends and family to honor the memory of his father. One day several weeks later, Jim was looking out of the car window as his mother was driving him to school and noticed the oak tree in the field. It occurred to him that he was moving on beyond the oak tree in the car, but that the oak tree stayed standing in the field as he moved. He described this observation to his mom. She was amazed at his insight. Gradually over the next few weeks the feeling of moving on gained momentum and eventually he looked forward to seeing the oak tree, and anticipated seeing it not with sadness but with a warm feeling. His life was opening up to new possibilities, his dad's memory increasingly was a comfort rather than a hole in his heart, and he felt relief and new energy. His mom had been able to transition into her new job, to be available to Jim, to ask for help from family and friends and to say yes when they offered. She was not yet able to imagine a renewed future for herself, but she was getting there.

REFERENCES

Aries, P. (1981). *The hour of our death.* New York: Alfred A. Knopf.

Attig, T. (1996). *How we grieve: Relearning the world.* New York: Oxford University Press.

Black, D. (1996). Childhood bereavement. *British Student Medical Journal,* 312, 1496-1500.

Bowlby, J. (1960). Separation anxiety. *International Journal of Psychoanalysis,* 42, 317-340.

Bowlby, J. (1961). Childhood mourning and its implications for psychiatry. *American Journal of Psychiatry,* 118, 481-498.

Bowlby, J. (1980). *Attachment and loss.* Volume 3: *Loss: Sadness and depression.* New York: Basic Books.

Brent, S.B. (1977). Puns, metaphors, and misunderstandings in a two-year-old's conception of death. *Omega: Journal of Death and Dying,* 8(4), 285-293.

Cooley, C.H. (1909[1962]). *Social organization.* New York: Schocken Books. Originally published by Charles Scribner's Sons.

DeSpelder, L. and Strickland, A.L. (2002). *The last dance: Encountering death and dying.* Boston, MA: McGraw-Hill Higher Education.

Dyregrov, A. (1991). *Grief in children: A handbook for adults.* London: Jessica Kingsley.

Freud, S. (1961). Mourning and melancholia. *Collected Papers.* Volume 4. New York: Basic Books.

Furman, E. (1974). *A child's parent's dies: Studies in childhood bereavement.* New Haven, CT: Yale University Press.

Gilligan, C. (1993). *In a different voice: Psychological theory and women's development,* Second edition. Cambridge, MA: Harvard University Press.

Goldman, L. (2000). *Breaking the silence.* Washington, DC: Taylor & Francis.

Gorer, G. (1967). *Death, grief and mourning.* Garden City, NY: Doubleday.

Hatter, B.S. (1996). Children and the death of a parent or grandparent. In C.A. Corr and D.M. Corr (Eds.), *Handbook of childhood death and bereavement* (pp. 431-439). New York: Springer Publishing Company.

Hurd, R.C. (1999). Adults view their childhood bereavement experiences. *Death studies,* 23, 17-41.

Ingles, R. (1980). St. Christopher's Hospice. In M.P. Hamilton and H.F. Reid (Eds.), *A hospice handbook: A new way to care for the dying* (pp. 45-56). Grand Rapids, MI: Eerdmans.

Kavanaugh, R. (1972). *Facing death.* Baltimore, MD: Penguin Books.

Klass, D. (1996). Grief in Eastern culture: Japanese ancestor worship. In D. Klass, P.R. Silverman, and S.L. Nickman (Eds.), *Continuing bonds: New understandings of grief* (pp. 59-70). Bristol, PA: Taylor & Francis.

Koocher, G.P. (1973). Childhood, death, and cognitive development. *Developmental Psychology,* 9(3), 369-375. Cited in L. DeSpelder and A.L. Strickland (2002). *The last dance: Encountering death and dying.* Boston, MA: McGraw-Hill Higher Education.

Kübler-Ross, E. (1969). *On death and dying.* New York: MacMillan Press.

Marrone, R. (1997). *Death, mourning and caring.* Pacific Grove, CA: Brooks/Cole.

Mead, G.H. (1934). *Mind, self, and society.* Chicago: University of Chicago Press.

Meyer, J.W. (1988). The social construction of the psychology of childhood: Some contemporary processes. In E.M. Hetherington, R.M. Lermer, and M. Perlmutter (Eds.), *Child development in a life-span perspective* (pp. 47-65). Hillsdale, NJ: Lawrence Erlbaum Associates.

Miller, J.B. (1986). *New psychology of women.* Boston: Beacon Press.

Mitford, J. (1963). *The American way of death.* New York: Simon & Schuster.

Neuberger, J. (1987). *Caring for dying people of different faiths.* London: Austin Cornish.

Nickman, S.L., Silverman, P.R., and Normand, C.L. (1998). Children's construction of a deceased parent: The surviving parent's contribution. *Journal of Orthopsychiatry,* 68, 126-134.

Normand, C.L., Silverman, P.R., and Nickman, S.L. (1996). Bereaved children's changing relationships with the deceased. In D. Klass, P.R. Silverman, and S.L. Nickman (Eds.), *Continuing bonds: New understandings of grief* (pp. 87-111). Bristol, PA: Taylor & Francis.

Parsons, T. (1994). Death in the western world. In R. Fulton and R. Bendickson (Eds.), *Death and identity* (pp. 60-79). Philadelphia: Charles Press.

Piaget, J. (1954). *The construction of reality in the child.* New York: Basic Books.

Rosenblatt, P.C. (1993). Grief: The social context of private feelings. In M.S. Stroebe, W. Stroebe, and R.O. Hansson (Eds.), *Handbook of bereavement* (pp. 102-111). New York: Cambridge University Press.

Rosenblatt, P.C., Walsh, R.P., and Jackson, D.A. (1976). *Grief and mourning in cross cultural perspective.* New Haven, CT: HRAF Press.

Sanders, C.M. (1995). Grief of children and parents. In K.J. Doka (Ed.), *Children mourning, mourning children* (pp. 69-84). Washington, DC: Hospice Foundation of America.

Schaeffer, D. and Lyons, D. (1993). *How do we tell the children?* New York: Newmarket.

Shapiro, E.R. (1994). *Grief as a family process: A developmental approach to clinical practice.* New York: The Guilford Press.

Silverman, P.R. (2000). *Never too young to know: Death in children's lives.* New York: Oxford University Press.

Silverman, P.R. and Klass, D. (1996). Introduction: What's the problem? In D. Klass, P.R. Silverman, and S.L. Nickman (Eds.), *Continuing bonds: New understandings of grief* (pp. 2-27). Bristol, PA: Taylor & Francis.

Silverman, P.R. and Worden, J.W. (1992). Children's reactions in the early months after the death of a parent. *American Journal of Orthopsychiatry, 62,* 93-104.

Stroebe, M. and Schut, H. (1999). The dual process model of coping with bereavement: Rationale and description. *Death Studies, 23,* 197-224.

Sullivan, H.S. (1972). *Personal psychopathology: Early formulations.* New York: Norton.

Titmuss, R. (1968). *Commitment to welfare.* New York: Pantheon Books.

Volkan, V.D. (1981). *Linking objects and linking phenomena.* New York: International Universities Press.

Wass, H. and Corr, C. (Eds.) (1984). *Childhood and death.* Washington, DC: Hemisphere.

Worden, J.W. (1991). *Grief counseling and grief therapy: A handbook for the mental health practitioner.* New York: Springer Publishing Company.

Worden, J.W. (1996). *Children and grief: When a parent dies.* New York: The Guilford Press.

Worden, J.W. and Silverman, P.S. (1996). Parental death and the adjustment of school-age children. *Omega, 33*(2), 91-102.

Chapter 7

Family Health Social Work Practice with Mexican Migrant and Seasonal Farmworking Families

Chrystal C. Ramirez Barranti

INTRODUCTION

My name is Jose Luis Rios, and I am in third grade. I have nine brothers and sisters. We live with our parents and aunt and uncle and cousins in Las Lomas. . . . All my relatives that I can think of work in the fields. . . . My parents work in la fresa [the strawberries] and la mora [the raspberries], and my mom sometimes packs mushrooms. Last year my father took me to the fields a lot during the week, too, instead of bringing me to school. I would find out I was going because he would say, "Let's go pick strawberries now." . . . My parents can't always find work. Usually there is work in the summer, so then I help my father every day in the fields. I have to pull up the grass around the strawberries, and I pick. I have to bend over. I bend over for a long time . . . but sometimes it is hard and I'm tired in school on Mondays because I worked on the weekend. I also get a lot of bad headaches, so sometimes I have to leave school early or go and rest in the nurse's office. When my father took me to the fields last year during the week, it was hard to study when I got home because I was tired. It is hard to work and go to school at the same time. (Atkin, 1993, pp. 11-15)

The author wishes to acknowledge the efforts of Dr. Christy Price of Dalton State College, Dalton, Georgia, and of Dr. Maria Dinis, Assistant Professor of Social Work, California State University, Sacramento. Tthese valued colleagues provided their invaluable expertise in the development of this chapter.

Mexican migrant and seasonal farmworking families are not an image of the past. They are mothers, fathers, brothers, sisters, aunts, uncles, cousins, nieces, nephews, grandmothers, and grandfathers who today are working together in America's farm fields. The economic hardship and abject poverty in which Mexican migrant and seasonal farmworking families live are not experiences of a hard-working people in the past, but shamefully is the continued plight of forgotten and invisible families.

It has been more than thirty years since Cesar Chavez courageously organized California's farmworkers and formed the United Farm Workers of America (UFW, n.d.) to fight for basic human rights, better wages, and humane working conditions for those who labored in the fields. Despite the great strides accomplished over the years, and the continued battles being waged by the United Farm Workers Union and other advocacy groups across the United States, the plight of the twenty-first century's migrant and seasonal farmworkers remains dismal. In fact, many who have documented the lives of migrant farmworkers in the United States found that conditions have instead worsened in recent years (Rothenberg, 1998).

Issues facing Mexican migrant and seasonal farmworkers and their families are found in every area of life, including prenatal development, health and disease, lack of safe housing, poor wages, hunger, dangerous working environments, and ineffectual immigration policies, to name only a few. Perhaps no other at-risk population in the United States suffers so greatly and overwhelmingly. Social injustice, prejudice, oppression, maltreatment, exploitation, and inequality are daily experiences of those who harvest fields (Human Rights Watch [HRW], 2000; Rothenberg, 1998).

Yet despite the glaring realities of migrant farmworking individuals and families, little has been written about social work practice and few, if any, social work journal articles concerning this vulnerable and at-risk group. This striking omission in the social work professional literature most definitely begs a call to action and advocacy. If the profession of social work is to continue to honorably embrace its mission, core values, and ethical principles, social workers must turn a bright light on the conditions of this population.

Perhaps it is within the framework of the family health social work practice model that social workers and other social service professionals can begin to answer this critical call to action and advocacy.

As Yuen (2003) emphasizes, "Family health social work practice places strong emphasis on working with populations that are at risk and affected by discrimination and oppression" (p. 26). This social work practice model clearly provides a good fit for understanding, assessing, and intervening with migrant farmworkers. In fact, given the multilevel vulnerability of Mexican migrant farmworking families, the family health social work practice model may significantly offer a helpful model for conceptualizing strengths, challenges, and problems as well as designing integrative multilevel interventions that enhance family health and well-being for farmworking families (Yuen, Skibinski, and Pardeck, 2003).

In order to support family health social work practice with Mexican migrant farmworking families, it is critical that practioners understand the transactional dynamics that occur within and between the ecological and systemic environment in which farmworking individuals and families habitate and develop their niches (Pardeck, 2003; Yuen, 2003).

It is fundamental that social workers using the family health perspective in their work with farmworking families gain a strong understanding of the dynamic biopsychosocial dimensions of farmworkers lives. For example, eight dimensions (economics, working conditions, housing, physical health and dental health, mental health and substance abuse, experiencing a migratory lifestyle, citizenship status, and culture and language) viewed through the theoretical lenses of ecological, systems, social constructionism, and developmental theories provide conceptual components of a holistic view of family health. In this approach, family health is defined well beyond the more common and narrower biomedical construct that relates only to physical disease and treatment. Rather, family health is conceptualized as a dynamic state of meaningful, multidimensional connections with persons and the environment in which the environment is inclusive of both the natural world as well as the socially constructed world (Pardeck and Yuen, 1999). More specifically, family health is defined by its crafters as

> a state of holistic well-being of the family system. Family health is manifested by the development of, and continuous interaction among, the physical, mental, emotional, social, economic, cultural, and spiritual dimensions of the family, which results in the

holistic well-being of the family and its members. (Pardeck and Yuen, 1999, p. 1)

The near invisibility of migrant farmworking families has left the details of their lives unknown to most people, including social workers. The first section of this chapter explores the ecological and systemic environments as well as the habitats and niches of Mexican migrant farmworking families. Throughout this discussion the reader will gain critical knowledge of the demographics of Mexican migrant and seasonal farmworking families. The ecological and systemic environments of farmworking families will be highlighted through discussion of the biospyschosocial dimensions that dynamically transact within the environments and between other ecosystems. Among the factors that impact and dynamically interact with Mexican migrant farmworking family health and well-being are economics, working conditions, housing, physical health and dental health, and mental health and substance abuse. Culture is identified within the family health social work practice model as a critical dimension of meaning and context. This, too, will be explored, along with citizenship status and language. Finally, the niche and habitat of the Mexican migrant farmworking family[1] as one of constant migration with the intent of making a living and providing for themselves and their families will be examined.

MY NAME IS COMPESINO

Mi Gente Son El Color de La Tierra
(My people are the color of the earth)
(Villaneuva, 1994, p. 314)

A key principle of the ecological perspective rests in recognizing that individuals, families, and groups are in dynamic transactions with their physical, social, political, and economic environments, all of which occurs within a dynamic cultural context (Germain and Gitterman, 1996). Understanding the critical dimensions and aspects that currently define Mexican migrant farmworkers and their families within the macroenvironment of the United States provides the practitioner with a springboard for implementing the family health social work practice model.

It is estimated that each year anywhere from 3 to 5 million farmworkers labor in the fields of America's farmlands (National Center for Farmworker Health [NCFH], 2002). Included among these are approximately 800,000 farmworking children (HRW, 2000). Since the early 1960s the farmworking population has been becoming increasingly Latino (Rothenberg, 1998). The National Center for Farmworker Health (2002) reports that at least 85 percent of all farmworkers working in the United States are Latino with a majority of them being Mexican or of Mexican descent.[2] There is great diversity within Mexico itself, and many Mexican immigrant migrant farmworkers are indigenous peoples such as the Miztecs, the Oaxacans, and the Zapotecas who speak indigenous languages (Bacon, 2002; Rothenberg, 1998).

America's farmworkers are categorized into two different groups: those who migrate and those who are referred to as seasonal farmworkers. Migrant farmworkers are those who do not return to their homes at the end of a day's hard work. They may be living in a migrant camp, sleeping under a tree, or living out of their car as they move from one harvest to another. Seasonal farmworkers, on the other hand, are defined as someone whose principal employment is in agriculture, works the fields seasonally, and has settled in one area where he or she returns home. Mexican immigrants are represented in both groups.

Migrant farmworking families follow three different geographic streams in their work to harvest the fields (HRW, 2000; NCFH, 2002). The West Coast stream begins in southern California and moves up through northern California, Oregon, and Washington. Many of the West Coast stream migrant farmworkers spend their winters in southern and central California. Those who follow the Midwestern stream may winter in Texas and begin following the crops west and north through Arizona, California, Colorado, Iowa, Illinois, Minnesota, Wisconsin, and Michigan. Following the fruit and vegetable harvests, migrant farmworkers in the Atlantic stream begin in Florida and work their way up through Georgia, the Carolinas, Maryland, New Jersey, New York, Maine, and eastern Michigan. As they travel virtually across the country, migrant farmworking families often go unnoticed—remaining invisible to the general public.

It is an appalling paradox that in the richest and most well-fed country in the world, those who work to bring food to America's tables are the poorest workers in the country. For example, a profile of migrant and seasonal farmworker families includes such facts as the following (Association of Farmworker Opportunity Programs [AFOP], 2002; Migrant and Seasonal Farmworker Children, 1998; Rothenberg, 1998):

- Average annual income is less than $7,500.
- The median educational level is six years of schooling.
- Two-thirds are thirty-five years old or younger.
- Sixty-six percent of farmworking parents have their children with them.
- Due to extreme poverty, children of migrant farmworkers often begin working the fields as young as age four.
- Forty percent of the children begin working in the fields at an average age of seven years old.
- More than half have emigrated from Mexico.
- About 60 percent are legally authorized to work in the United States.
- Nationally, nearly 40 percent are undocumented.
- Eighty percent do not speak English. Spanish or other indigenous languages are their primary languages.
- Life expectancy of a farmworker is forty-nine years of age.

This composite view of Mexican migrant farmworkers depicts vulnerable populations who live in extreme poverty, have poor health, and experience overwhelming psychosocial and sociopolitical barriers that compromise individual and family health and well-being. This composite provides a description of the larger habitat and niche occupied by Mexican migrant and seasonal farmworking families. The next section zooms in for a closer look at the ecological and systemic environments, which are highlighted through discussion of several biospyschosocial dimensions that dynamically transact with one another within the environments and between other ecosystems of Mexican migrant farmworking families.

BIOPSYCHOSOCIAL DIMENSIONS IMPACTING
WELL-BEING AND FAMILY HEALTH

Increasing the understanding of the ecology of farmworking families requires a close examination of several critical biopsychosocial dimensions that contribute to how Mexican migrant farmworking families come to occupy a particular habitat and define their niche. Before exploring the individual dimensions, it is helpful to provide a definition of both habitat and niche. According to Germain and Gitterman (1996), a *habitat* is defined as an individual's, family's, or group's physical and social settings. Habitats that are supportive of health and well-being provide community resources that are available and accessible to all living in the habitat. On the other hand, "habitats that do not support the growth, health, and social functioning of individuals and families . . . are likely to produce isolation, disorientation, and helplessness" (Germain and Gitterman, 1996, p. 20).

Niche is defined as the position or status that the individual, family, and/or group occupies within the social structure of the habitat (Germain and Gitterman, 1996). Similar to habitats, niches can be supportive, enhancing health and well-being. Since the niche of a particular family or group is influenced by sociopolitical and economic social structures as well as access to societal rights, some niches are unsupportive of growth and well-being (Germain and Gitterman, 1996). "Such niches are shaped and sustained by society's tolerance of the misuse of power in political, social, and economic structures" (Germain and Gitterman, 1996, p. 20).

What elements of the ecological environment influence and shape migrant farmworking families' habitat and niche? The following looks again at some of the dimensions that contribute to defining the habitat and niche of Mexican migrant farmworking families:

- economics,
- working conditions,
- housing,
- physical health and dental health,
- mental health and substance abuse,
- experiencing of a migratory lifestyle,
- citizenship status, and
- culture and language.

Economics

Mexican migrant farmworking families occupy a niche in U.S. society that is of great value yet promotes invisibility and marginalization. That is, migrant farmworking families make a significant contribution to the U.S. economy as they are literally the muscle behind the multibillion-dollar agricultural industry (NCFH, 2002). A critical contributing force to America's quality of life, farmworkers are responsible for harvesting every piece of fruit and every vegetable that fill our grocery stores and grace our dining tables. Yet despite this crucial and invaluable niche, farmworking families are exploited by a farm-labor system that keeps them in extreme poverty (HRW, 2000; Rothenberg, 1998).

Mexican migrant and seasonal farmworking families are among the poorest and the most neglected in our nation. In fact, they earn the lowest wages of any occupational group in the United States. Average annual earnings are approximately $7,500 for seasonal farmworkers, and migrant farmworking families earn less than $5,000 a year (NCFH, 2002; Rothenberg, 1998). However, those migrant farmworkers who come to the fields through a farm-labor contractor earn even less, averaging about $3,500 annually (Rothenberg, 1998). It is not surprising then that, despite the many family members who work in the fields, more than two-thirds of farmworker families live well below the poverty line and most fall at least 100 percent below the federal poverty level (Arendale, 2001; Rothenberg, 1998).

The extreme poverty in which migrant farmworker families live often requires a whole-family effort toward generating an income. Many families struggle with the decision to bring their children into the fields to work. Children work at the expense of their own education, health, and social development (Atkin, 1993; Gwyther and Jenkins, 1998; HRW, 2000). Agriculture is the only occupation in which children under age sixteen are allowed to work (HRW, 2000). It is not uncommon for children as young as four years old to be working alongside their parents. Full-time farmwork can begin in early adolescence, between the ages of thirteen years and fifteen years (Atkin, 1993; Gwyther and Jenkins, 1998; HRW, 2000). Under the Fair Labor Standards Act (U.S. General Accounting Office, 1998), farmworker children and youth are the least protected of all U.S. laborers. For example, no standards are set for how many hours migrant children can work. Fourteen- to eighteen-hour days and seven-day workweeks are not uncommon during peak harvest in seasons (HRW, 2000). Most children earn well under minimum wage and do not get overtime pay.

Jessica G., for example, left school two years ago at the age of fifteen to work in the melon fields near Yuma, where the season runs from November to April. She worked from 4:00 am until 3:00 or 4:00 pm—an eleven- or twelve-hour day. She earned $36 a day—at about $3.00 an hour—well below minimum wage. "It's very difficult work," she said. "You're outside all day, with just a few short breaks. I was very tired at the end of the day." Both the manager of the farm and the farm-labor contractor who hired Jessica G. were friends of her family. Four of the five children in Jessica G.'s family have worked in the fields. Jessica's grandmother raised the children, as their mother always worked in the fields. (HRW, 2000, p. 39)

Although strides have been made by such groups as the UFW to increase hourly and piecework wages, migrant and seasonal farmworkers have actually lost economic ground in the past decade because salaries have decreased in real wages by 5 percent (NCFH, 2002). In addition to the impact of lost wages through the drop in real wages, farmworking families are extremely vulnerable to wage exploitation (HRW, 2000; Rothenberg, 1998). Wage rates promised may not be honored or earned wages may not be paid at all. In fact, some crew leaders and labor contractors outright take their farmworkers money (HRW, 2000; Rothenberg, 1998). Financial exploitation also occurs when employers do not report or underreport wages paid to farmworkers, the result if which is no Social Security, disability, or retirement benefits (HRW, 2001; NCFH, 2002).

Working Conditions

In 1989, farmwork was classified as the most dangerous work in the country, surpassing even mining (National Safety Council [NSC], 1989). Those who work in the fields are exposed to significant amounts of pesticides, fertilizers, and other biohazards. Farmwork requires the use of heavy and dangerous machinery, vehicles, and farmworking tools. Needless to say, farmworkers perform hard physical labor for long hours in the sun and heat, sometimes without enough potable water or the availability of lavatories (HRW, 2000). In fact, farms with ten or fewer workers are legally exempt from having to provide toilets, handwashing facilities, or drinking water. Some farmers and farm-labor contractors actually charge farmworkers for drinking water (HRW, 2000; Rothenberg, 1998). Farms with eleven or more workers need only provide toilets, handwashing facilities, and drinking water within one-quarter mile of the work site. Shamefully, the enforcement of sanitation, potable water, and handwashing facilities is often neglected in some states (HRW, 2000; Bechtel, Davidhizar, and Spurlock, 2000; Bechtel, Shepherd, and Rogers, 1995).

Art Morelos, a top official of the Occupational Safety and Health Division Of the Industrial Commission of Arizona—often referred to as "state OSHA" or "Arizona OSHA"—told Human Rights Watch that a lack of toilets was, together with a lack of drinking cups, the "biggest complaint in the fields" (HRW, 2000, p. 24). Notwithstanding this, the same official also reported that his agency, which is responsible for enforcing state sanitation regulations, does not do farm inspections on its own initiative and does not do surprise inspections.

Farmworking children and adolescents are likewise exposed to backbreaking and dangerous working conditions. Farmwork is rated as the most dangerous occupation in the United States (NSC, 1989), and it has also been rated as the most dangerous occupation in which children and adolescents are allowed to work (HRW, 2000). Children and adolescents are more vulnerable to risk of farmwork-related injuries than adults because of their lack of experience, their developing bodies, and their developing cognitive skills (HRW, 2000; AFOP, 2002). It is estimated that, annually, 100,000 farmworking children and adolescents suffer some kind of farmworking injury (National Research Council and Institute of Medicine [1998] as cited in HRW, 2000).

Housing: No Place Like Home

Migrant farmworking families have a very difficult time finding adequate housing or housing at all. More often than not, when housing is found, it is substandard, unsafe, and lacking in proper sanitation (Holden, 2001). One statewide study discovered in the process of the survey that when asking about their current housing situations, the range of responses included, "house, apartment, trailer, motor home, tool shed, garage, tent, and automobile" (Villarejo et al., 2000, p. 11).

ESTELA: When we first arrived, we started looking for work. We ended up in Stockton, picking cherries.

ANTONIO: We spent three weeks there, sleeping under the trees, out in the open air. We spread blankets and sheets on the ground and cooked over a fire.

ESTELA: Then we went to Oregon.

ANTONIO: At the ranchero where we worked, there were over a hundred people. Like in Stockton, we all slept outside. In the afternoon it would get cold. There were no showers and no hot water. To bathe we had to fill up a bucket with water and go out into the orchard. Many people brought children. When we saw this, we thought about going back home. (Rothenberg, 1998, p. 22)

The Housing Assistance Council (HAC, 2001) recently sponsored a nationwide study of farmworker housing to help determine current living conditions and housing needs of migrant farmworking families (HAC, 2001). The study included surveys of more than 4,600 dwellings in which migrant farmwokers were living. Fifty-two percent were crowded (having more than one person to a room) and, of these, 74 percent had children. Overcrowding and sharing residential space is a direct result of low incomes and the inability to afford even the least costly of rentals.

In addition to overcrowding, many dwellings were found to be unsafe and unsanitary, often without an essential working appliance such as a stove or refrigerator. The location of available housing or living areas often placed migrant farmworking families in direct exposure to pesticides and other biochemical hazards. More than 26 percent of the dwellings in the study were directly alongside pesticide-treated fields, placing children remaining at home in direct exposure. Functioning bathing facilities, laundry facilities, or both were found to be lacking in 53 percent of these residential areas, increasing the impact of exposure. Additional substandard conditions included serious structural deficiencies such as sagging roofs, porches, and house frames; foundation damage; broken windows; holes in the roof, floors, and walls; peeling paint; broken plaster; exposed wiring; and leaks.

Substandard and unsafe housing has a direct relation to serious health problems (Holden, 2001). Overcrowding has been associated with increased incidence of infectious diseases such as tuberculosis. Hepatitis and pesticide poisoning have been linked to lack of proper sanitation, broken appliances, and contaminated drinking water. Exposure to pesticides, molds, rodent infestations, and insects contribute to respiratory diseases such as asthma. Peeling paint that is lead based has resulted in lead poisoning among migrant children, resulting in serious long-term damage.

Physical space is a significant element of the life space that influences health and well-being. When a physical space does not support such human needs as safety, comfort, and family life, it affords additional biopsychosocial stresses. A family's home is considered the physical space in which members are nurtured, food is prepared, rest takes place, children study, and members spend time together. The inadequate housing conditions experienced by migrant farmworking families presents not only serious physical safety issues, but exacerbates already overwhelming stressors.

Health and Dental Health: A Third World Picture

The average life span of a farmworker in the United States is forty-nine years (NCFH, 2002). This is a startling if not shocking fact, especially when viewed against the average life span 76.9 years for the general public (Centers for Disease Control and Prevention [CDC], 2002). The complexity of health problems experienced by farmworking families is a result of dangerous working conditions that assault almost every organ of one's body, extreme poverty, poor nutrition, lack of access to health care, and the inability to afford medical treatment.

The health problems of farmworkers and their children are more complex than those of the general public. Adults and children suffer more frequently from infectious diseases of all types, including tuberculosis, hepatitis, and viral, bacterial, and fungal illnesses. It is not uncommon for farmworking families to suffer from intestinal parasites (Bechtel, 1998). Exposure to deficient sanitation and contaminated drinking water at the work site and housing sites are often the contributing causes for these diseases (Ciesielski et al., 1992; Larson, 2001; Wilk, 1993).

Farmwork has been rated by National Safety Council (1989) as the most hazardous occupation. It is no wonder that working in the fields places migrant farmworking families in harm's way—exposing them to the danger of severe occupational injuries. Musculoskeletal injuries from heavy lifting, repetitive movements, poor or broken equipment, and long work hours have resulted in chronic conditions and disabilities (Larson, 2001; Villarejo and Baron, 1999). Devastating injuries such as crushing from farm equipment, falls, cuts, amputations, and resulting fatalities are not uncommon in farmwork (Bureau of Labor Statistics, 2000). Migrant farmworker children and youth are not exempt from exposure to danger or from injury (Bechtel et al., 2000; HRW, 2000; NCFH, 2001).

Although working among large and dangerous machinery places farmworking families at risk for debilitating injuries and, at times, fatalities, perhaps the most insidious agricultural hazard is exposure to pesticides and fertilizers (Larson, 2001; Von Essen and McCurdy, 1998). In fact, more than 300,000 farmworkers are poisoned annually (Gwyther and Jenkins, 1998; Larson, 2001; NCFH, 2002). Such exposure results in myriad illnesses significantly affecting family health and well-being (HRW, 2000; Larson, 2001; NCFH, 2002). High rates of chronic respiratory diseases such as asthma and bronchitis are directly related to chemical and fertilizer exposures. In addition, pesticide exposure has been linked to spontaneous abortions, birth defects, and sterility. Such exposure also results in severe cancers of the brain, breast cancers, non-Hodgkin's lymphoma, leukemia, and skin cancers. Neurological damage has also resulted from exposure to chemicals and biological materials:

> On June 27, 1992, seventeen-year-old migrant farmworker Jose Antonio Casillas collapsed and died while riding his bike near his home in rural Utah. Emergency workers found foam streaming from his nose. According to Jose's uncle, the day before he died, the boy had been soaked with pesticide sprayed from a tractor; a week earlier he had also been sprayed, while working in a peach orchard. After the second spraying he showed symptoms of severe pesticide poisoning, including vomiting, sweating, diarrhea and headaches. He had received no training from his employer regarding pesticide dangers and the symptoms of exposure, and reportedly slept in his pesticide-soaked clothing the night before his death. (HRW, 2000, p. 17)

While occupation-related illnesses, injuries, and diseases are significant contributors to the complexity of health issues experienced by migrant and seasonal farmworking families, the impact of destitute poverty itself adds an additional vulnerability to health and well-being. Poverty-related illnesses include such infectious diseases as tuberculosis, parasites, diabetes, and HIV/AIDS (Bechtel, 1998; Organista, Organista, and Soloff, 1998).

Despite that farmworking families harvest the food that feeds the nation, malnutrition among farmworking families is rampant (Gwyther and Jenkins, 1998). Poor nutrition results in pre- and postpartum infant deaths, anemia, severe dental problems, and poor mental and physical development. The infant mortality rate among farmworking families is 25 percent higher than the national average (NCFH, 2001, 2002). Birth injuries are not uncommon and have been found to include cerebral palsy and mental retardation.

Dental and oral health has been identified as one of the top five health problems for migrant and seasonal farmworkers from age five through age twenty-nine years (Lombardi, 2001). It ranks among the top twenty for other farmworker age groups. In fact, farmworker dental decay is found to be twice that of the general population in the United States. Similarly, the incidence of baby bottle tooth decay occurs at about a 10 percent greater incidence than that found among the children of the urban poor (Lombardi, 2001).

Barriers to Health Care

The overall health and well-being of migrant and seasonal farmworking families is reflective of what is found in third world agrarian societies (Bechtel, Davidhizar, and Spurlock, 2000). Although federally funded migrant health centers are found in agricultural areas of the nation, they have been able to reach only about 15 percent of all migrant and seasonal farmworkers annually (Bechtel, Shepherd, and Rogers, 1995). Dental and oral health components of the migrant health centers have been underfunded, understaffed, or do not have a dentist on staff (Lombardi, 2001). In many rural areas there is simply a lack of available health care and dental health care providers. Potential clinics may be far from the work site or the migrant camp and the lack of transportation often prevents farmworkers from accessing distant health or dental care sites (Bechtel, Davidhizar, and Spurlock,

2000; Gwyther and Jenkins, 1998; Lombardi, 2001). Commonly, no money may be available to pay for treatment. Taking time off of work to see a doctor or to recover from illness or injury is unthinkable because of the severe loss of wages.

Language and cultural health beliefs and assumptions are also barriers for Mexican migrant farmworking families, as too often health care providers do not have an understanding of the Spanish language or other indigenous dialects (Bechtel, Shepherd, and Rogers, 1995; Betchel, Davidhizar, and Spurlock, 2000). A lack of knowledge by health care providerse about culturally related beliefs and assumptions about health and medical care has also been found to be a barrier (Bechtel, Shepherd, and Rogers, 2000; Larson, 2001; Lombardi, 2001).

Migratory life with its continuous movement makes consistent medical care and follow-up care very difficult if not impossible (Bechtel, Shepherd, and Rogers, 1995; Betchel, Davidhizar, and Spurlock, 2000; Gwyther and Jenkins, 1998). Similar to many of the working poor in this country, farmworking families very rarely have any kind of health insurance (Arendale, 2001; NCFH, 2002). For example, the California Agricultural Worker Health Survey (Villarejo et al., 2000) found that only one-third of the 971 migrant and seasonal farmworkers they surveyed had any form of health insurance. Only 7 percent reported being enrolled in government-offered insurance programs such as Medicaid and the State Child's Health Insurance Program (Lombardi, 2001).

Mental Health and Substance Abuse

The economics, working and housing conditions, and health status of migrant and seasonal farmworking families presents a picture of life that is tremendously overwhelming. Certainly the environmental stressors previously identified could be enough to place any individual at risk for mental health and substance abuse problems. Recognizing the potential vulnerability of migrant farmworkers to mental health problems and substance abuse research has recently begun (Alderete et al., 2000; De Leon Siantz, 1994; Hovey, 2001; Hovey and Magana, 2000). From this research, Hovey (2001) has identified a set of stressors frequently experienced by migrant and seasonal farmworking families which place them at risk for depression, anxiety, suicide, and substance abuse.

The research exploring the mental health status of migrant farmworkers has tapped subjects from different migrant streams. For example, a Texas study of Mexican migrant mothers found that 41 percent of the women met diagnostic criteria for depression (De Leon Siantz, 1994). Among Mexican migrant farmworkers in Michigan and Ohio, 38 percent were found to be clinically depressed (Hovey and Magana, 2000). Finally, a Fresno County, California, study documented that 20 percent of the Mexican migrant farmworkers studied had symptomology that met the diagnosis for depression (Alderete et al., 2000). Significant risk factors for depression among Mexican migrant farmworkers include

- lack of support from family and friends,
- high acculturative stress,
- low religiosity,
- low self-esteem,
- lower income,
- lack of child care,
- higher levels of education,
- lack of empowerment to control one's life, and
- discrimination.

The Mexican culture has many qualities that contribute to family resiliency in the face of significant stress (Falicov, 1998). Such cultural dimensions as family relationships, the significance of affiliation and social relationships, and an orientation to collectivist values have been found to be effective buffers protecting Mexican migrant farmworking families from depression (Alderete et al., 2000; Hovey, 2001). When there is an absence of emotional and/or instrumental support from family and friends, risk for depression among Mexican migrant farmworkers increases (De Leon Siantz, 1994; Hovey, 2001; Hovey and Magana, 2000).

Suicide risk is a realistic possibility for those who are experiencing depression, yet almost nothing is known about suicide and suicidiality among migrant farmworking families (Hovey, 2001). A small study of twenty Mexican migrant farmworking mothers in Michigan and Ohio found that 35 percent reported a history of suicidal thought

(Hovey and Magana, 2000). Out of this study, several suicidal risk factors that may contribute to the vulnerability of migrant farmworking mothers' vulnerability to suicidal ideation were identified to include low self-esteem, lack of social support, increased hopelessness about the future, greater acculturative stress, dysfunctional family system, and higher levels of depression.

Although the research on depression and suicide among migrant farmworking families is scant, even less research exists on the prevalence of anxiety (Hovey, 2001). A Fresno County, California, study (Alderete et al., 2000) of Mexican migrant farmworkers found that 15.1 percent of the men and 12.9 percent of the women had experienced an anxiety disorder during their lifetime. The Michigan and Ohio studies (Hovey, 2001) found that 29.5 percent had symptoms of overall anxiety (affective and cognitive) indicating that migrant farmworkers are at risk for developing anxiety disorders (Hovey, 2001). A number of risk factors unique to the lives of Mexican migrant farmworker families also create vulnerabilities to anxiety and anxiety disorders (Alderete et al., 2000; Hovey, 2001). These factors include ineffective social support, high acculturative stress, low religiosity, low self-esteem, nonimmigrant status, and female gender.

Alcohol and drugs are used by many populations to easily self-medicate stressful or painful conditions. Migrant farmworkers are no different in their use of substances as a means of coping with depression, anxiety, loneliness, discrimination, oppression, and the hardships of poverty (HRW, 2000; Mines, Mullenax, and Saca, 2001; Perilla, 1998). In addition, some farmworker youth and younger farmworkers use amphetamines to help them work faster and for long hours (HRW, 2000).

A California study found alcoholism to be more prevalent than other psychiatric diagnoses among the men (Alderete et al., 2000). Another study found that two-thirds of Mexican migrant farmworkers drank, and of those who consumed alcohol, 75 percent were men and 11 percent were women (Mines, Mullenax, and Saca, 2001). They typically drank two days per week and had three drinks per sitting. Thirteen percent indicated that they drank six to seven days per week and about twenty-one drinks per week. The effects of alcohol and substance abuse on health, mental health, the family, one's social relationships, and work are well documented (Johnson, 2003). Given the high danger involved in farmwork, alcohol and substance abuse among farmworkers also places using farmworkers at greater risk for injury (Alaniz, 1994).

Experiencing a Migratory Life

Mexican migrant farmworking families live and work within a complex set of major stressors such as extreme poverty, dangerous work, unwelcoming sociopolitical environments, lack of access to health and social services, and, at times, separation from family and friends. The impact of such major life-sphere stressors on family well-being and health is intensified when realized within the context and experience of migration itself.

The very experience of migration is considered to be a risk to health and well-being. As migrant farmworking families follow the harvesting of crops, they live in a cycle of constant uprooting and re-settling. A sense of instability and anxiety often comes with moving to the next harvest. Frequently there is no guarantee of work or housing at the new site. The reality of discrimination, oppression, and prejudice adds to anticipatory anxiety when entering potentially unwelcoming communities.

Geographic and social isolation is frequently a consequence of a migratory life. For example, most migrant camps are located next to the fields in remote areas. Whereas some Mexican migrant farmworking families migrate with members of their extended family, others can be cut off from extended family and social support networks. This can be especially true for Mexican immigrants whose families remain in Mexico.

Parents worry about the impact of moving on their children's social development and education (Duarte and Rafanello, 2001; Gwyther and Jenkins, 1998; Henning-Stout, 1996). The cumulative effect of continuous mobility, poverty, and working long hours in the fields often means exhaustion, absenteeism, and the loss of friends and social groups. Not only can migrant children and youth struggle with discouragement, but they are also at high risk for depression, anxiety, and behavior problems (Kupersmidt and Martin, 1997). It may not be surprising then to find that the national dropout rate for migrant farmworker youth is 45 percent (HRW, 2000).

The effects of living in such a nonnutritive environment does not result solely in mental illness, substance abuse, and poor health.

Other indicators that a family's health and well-being are at risk exist as well. Collapsing under overwhelming stressors, some migrant farmworking families can find themselves involved in domestic violence, child neglect/abuse, and divorce (HRW, 2000; Larson, Doris, and Alvarez, 1990; Rodriguez, 2001; Rothenberg, 1998).

Citizenship Status

Citizenship status is an important factor when considering the context of Mexican migrant farmworking families. Those who work the fields and are undocumented carry an extra burden of stress. The work of remaining invisible so as not to be caught and deported heightens anxiety and almost always requires a level of social isolation (Falicov, 2002; Hovey, 2001). Consequently, loneliness and fear are often common emotional companions for those who are undocumented. Documentation status is an important factor when considering access to health and social services. Living without documentation is often a barrier to seeking and receiving needed services because to access services can mean deportation (Gutierrez, Yeakly, and Ortega, 2000; HRW, 2000).

Culture and Language

Although the previous explanations depict poverty, poor health, and other barriers to individual well-being, it is important to note that despite severe challenges, the Mexican migrant and seasonal farmworking family is resilient and has many strengths from which to draw (Falicov, 1998, 2002; Hovey, 2001). Among these are family connectedness, physical and psychological presence of extended family, family rituals, spiritual belief systems, a strong work ethic, determination, tenacity, and a commitment to give their children a better life (Falicov, 2002). Such strengths are rooted in the Mexican culture, which is imbued with defining values. Defining cultural values provide a kaleidoscopic lens through which the world is viewed and experienced, and through which life is lived. The general cultural values that are characteristic of the Mexican culture include the following (Falicov, 1998, 2002; Gutierrez, Yeakley, and Ortega, 2000):

- family is primary,
- traditional gender roles,
- collective orientation,
- intergroup and intragroup harmony,
- direct confrontation and conflict are to be avoided,
- closeness in interpersonal space,
- present time orientation,
- spiritual orientation, and
- strong work ethic.

Understanding general cultural values and worldviews provides a general guide for understanding and relating with Mexican migrant farmworkers. Although there are general cultural values, diversity exists within each individual and for each unique family. In reality, individuals and families are defined by multiple cultural identities that include national region, language/dialect, gender, religion, social class, education, occupation, immigration experiences, and individual life stories (Falicov, 1998, 2002):

Noting both the general cultural values while recognizing the diversity within the unique individual and family, family health intervention strategies can be implemented that respect and build on the cultural values and inherent strengths of Mexican migrant farmworking families. For example, the family is primary in the Mexican culture in general and exceptionally significant in the lives of Mexican migrant families (Bechtel, Shepherd, and Rogers, 1995; Betchel, Davidhizar, and Spurlock, 2000; Gwyther and Jenkins, 1998; HRW, 2000; Rothenberg, 1998). Every family member makes an important contribution to the family's well-being by working in the fields and generating income, taking care of younger siblings or elders, translating for parents, and completing an education (Atkin, 1993; Bechtel, Davidhizar, and Spurlock, 2000).

A Mexican child has a very different sense of the importance of family than do many American children. Mexican children speak with respect about their grandparents and parents and most children want to contribute to their family somehow. They help by working and caring for the younger children. Because parents work in the fields and often have little education, they rely on their older children to help the younger ones in school and be positive role models. Because the needs of the family are stressed more than those of the individual, parents trust that when their children improve their lives, the whole family will benefit. (Atkin, 1993, p. 47)

Culture has a defining influence on the processes of communication. The collective orientation that is central in Mexican culture is inherently woven throughout all communication (Falicov, 1998, 2000). Relationships are highly valued, and the needs of the family and extended family take precedence over individual needs. Likewise, the cultural value of *personissmo* stresses the primacy of developing a personal relationship before a working relationship is begun, and the value of *respeto* highlights the significance of social hierarchy in the Mexican culture (Green, 1998; Gutierrez, Yeakley, and Ortega, 2000). The significance of maintaining harmony in relationships can be expressed through the hesitation to question or confront others, especially those who are considered to hold a higher position in the social hierarchy (Bechtel, Shepherd, and Rogers, 1995).

The language of a culture provides a view into the contextual meaning of communication. Yet meaning and connection can be lost if the primary language spoken is not the dominant language of one's living and working environment. Many Mexican migrant farmworking families speak only Spanish, and still many others speak an indigenous language such as Zapotec. Children are often the first to become bilingual and play a critical role in helping their parents bridge the language gap (Bechtel, Shepherd, and Rogers, 1995; Bechtel, Davidhizal, and Spurlock, 2000, 2000).

Traditionally, the orientation of the Mexican culture is toward present time (Green, 1998). The influence of time orientation in the lives of Mexican migrant farmworking families is a focus on the here and now. Intertwined with the pressures of poverty, the necessity of migration, and a very strong work ethic, the present-time orientation often supports the difficult decision to pull children from school to work in the fields as well as uproot children from school to follow the harvests (Bechtel, Shepherd, and Rogers, 1995). The idea of any kind of preventive health care or follow-up is lost when faced with the harsh realities of extreme poverty and the imperative to migrate for work (Bechtel, Shepherd, and Rogers, 1995).

Health beliefs are significantly influenced by one's culture and individual specific qualities such as social class, education, age, historical cohort membership, region of origin (rural, urban, etc.), spirituality, and whether a member of an indigenous people (Applewhite, 1996; Keegan, 1996; Lynch and Hanson, 1998). Mexican folk medicine can be an important cultural element for some Mexican migrant farmworkers. Within the tradition of Mexican folk medicine, healing is sought from such folk healers as *curanderos/curanderas* (folk healers), *yerberos* (herbalists), *hueseros* (bone specialists), *sobadores* (muscle specialists, masseurs), and *parteras* (midwives) (Applewhite, 1996). The focus of treatment can be spiritual, mental, and/or physical, and involves elements of faith and spirituality. Mexican folk healing is often used as an alternative to Western medicine and just as often in conjunction with it (Keegan, 1996).

CONCLUSION

Significant biospychosocial and environmental factors that impact the niche and habitat of Mexican migrant farmworking families were explored in this chapter. Understanding the elements that comprise the person-in-environment fit for migrant farmworking families is an important knowledge base for utilizing the family health social work practice model with migrant farmworkers. The chapter's inquiry into the person-in-environment dynamics of migrant farmworkers revealed a nonnutritive environment unsupportive of health and well-being. Social workers practicing from the family health social work model are oriented toward recognizing and building on the incredible resilience and strengths of a people who harvest fields through collaborative assessment and empowering intervention. The family health social work practice model is an especially applicable model that can enable the profession of social work to answer the call to advocacy and intervention with this vulnerable and terribly underserved people. As Cesar Chavez said, "Si se puede!" (Yes, we can!) (United Farmworkers of America, n.d.).

NOTES

1. Throughout this chapter the phrase *Mexican migrant farmworking families* will be used interchangeably with *migrant farmworking families* and *farmworking families.*

2. Although the focus of this chapter is the Mexican farmworkers, the author wishes to acknowledge that many other ethnocultures and nationalities also labor in the fields.

REFERENCES

Alaniz, M. L. (1994). Mexican farmworker women's perspectives on drinking in a migrant community. *The International Journal of the Addictions, 29,* 1173-1188.

Alderete, E., Vega, W. A., Kolody, B., and Aguilar-Gaxiola, S. (2000). Lifetime prevalence of and risk factors for psychiatric disorders among Mexican migrant farmworkers in California. *American Journal of Public Health, 90,* 608-614.

Applewhite, S. L. (1996). Curanderismo: Demystifying the health beliefs and practices of elderly Mexican American. In P. Ewalt, E. Freeman, S. Kirk, and D. Poole (Eds.), *Multicultural issues in social work* (pp. 455-468). Washington, DC: NASW Press.

Arendale, E. (2001). *Medicaid and the state children's health insurance program.* Migrant Health Issues: Monograph Series No 3. Buda, TX: National Center for Farmworker Health.

Association of Farmworker Opportunity Programs (AFOP) (2002). *Children in the fields: The inequitable treatment of child farmworkers* Available online at <www.afop.org/child_labor>.

Atkin, B. S. (1993). *Voices from the fields: Children of migrant farmworkers tell their stories.* Boston: Little, Brown and Company.

Bacon, D. (2002). *Binational Oaxacan indigenous migrant organizers face new century.* Americas Program, Silver City, NM: Interhemispheric Resource Center. Available online at <www.americaspolicy.org/articles/2002/0208oaxaca_body.html>.

Bechtel, G. A. (1998). Parasitic infections among migrant farm families. *Journal of Community Health Nursing, 15*(1), 1-7.

Bechtel, G. A., Davidhizar, R., and Spurlock, W. R. (2000). Migrant farm workers and their families: Cultural patterns and delivery of care in the United States. *International Journal of Nursing Practice, 6,* 300-306.

Bechtel, G. A., Shepherd, M. A., and Rogers, P. W. (1995). Family, culture, and health practices among migrant farmworkers. *Journal of Community Health Nursing, 12*(1), 15-22.

Bureau of Labor Statistics (2000). *Workplace injuries and illnesses in 1999.* Washington, DC: Author.

Centers for Disease Control and Prevention (CDC) (2002). Table 12. Estimated life expectancy at birth in years, by race and sex: Death-registration states, 1900-28, and United States, 1929-2000 [Electronic version]. *National Vital Statistics Reports, 51*(3). Available online at <www.cdc.gov/nchs>.

Ciesielski, S., Seed, J. R., Ortiz, J., and Metts, J. (1992). Intestinal parasites among North Carolina migrant farmworkers. *American Journal of Public Health, 82*(9), 1258-1262.

De Leon Siantz, M. L. (1994). The Mexican-American migrant farmworker family: Mental health issues. *Mental Health Nursing, 29*, 65-72.

Duarte, G. and Rafanello, D. (2001). The migrant child: A special place in the field. *Young Children, 56*(2), 26-34.

Falicov, C. J. (1998). *Latino families in therapy: A guide to multicultural practice.* New York: Guilford Press.

Falicov, C. J. (2002). Ambiguous loss: Risk and resilience in Latino immigrant families. In M. M. Suarez-Orozco and M. M. Paez (Eds.), *Latinos remaking America* (pp. 274-288). Berkeley, CA: University of California Press.

Germain, C. and Gitterman, A. (1996). *The live model of social work practice: Advances in theory and practice,* Second edition. New York: Columbia University Press

Green, J. (1998). *Cultural awareness in the human services.* Englewood Cliffs, NJ: Prentice Hall.

Gutierrez, L., Yeakley, A., and Ortega, R. (2000). Educating students for social work with Latinos: Issues for the new millennium. *Journal of Social Work Education, 36*(3), 541-557.

Gwyther, M. E. and Jenkins, M. (1998). Migrant farmworker children: Health status, barriers to care, and nursing innovations in health care delivery. *Journal of Pediatric Health Care, 12*(March/April), 60-66.

Henning-Stout, M. (1996). Que podemos hacer?: Roles for school psychologists with Mexican and Latino migrant children and families. *School Psychology Review, 25*(2), 154-164.

Housing Assistance Council (2001). *No refuge from the fields: Findings from a survey of farmworker housing in the United States.* Washington, DC: Author.

Holden (2001). *Housing.* Migrant Health Issues: Monograph Series No 8. Buda, TX: National Center for Farmworker Health.

Hovey, J. (2001). *Mental health and substance abuse.* Migrant Health Issues: Monograph Series No 4. Buda, TX: National Center for Farmworker Health.

Hovey, J. D. and Magana, C. (2000). Acculturative stress, anxiety, and depression among Mexican immigrant farmworkers in the Midwest United States. *Journal of Immigrant Health, 2,* 119-131.

Human Rights Watch (HRW) (2000). *Fingers to the bone: United States failure to protect child farmworkers.* New York: Author.

Johnson, J. L. (2003). *Fundamentals of substance abuse practice.* Belmont, CA: Wadsworth.

Keegan, L. (1996). Use of alternative therapies among Mexican Americans in the Texas Rio Grande Valley. *Journal of Holistic Health, 14*(4), 277-294.

Kupersmidt, J. B. and Martin, S. L. (1997). Mental health problems of children of migrant and seasonal farmworkers: A pilot study. *Child Abuse and Neglect, 36,* 224-232.

Larson, A. (2001). *Environmental/occupation safety and health.* Migrant Health Issues: Monograph Series No 2. Buda, TX: National Center For Farmworker Health.

Larson, D., Doris, J., and Alvarez, W. (1990). Migrants and maltreatment: Comparative evidence from central register data. *Child Abuse and Neglect, 14,* 375-385.

Lombardi, G. R (2001). *Dental/oral health services.* Migrant Health Issues: Monograph Series No 1. Buda, TX: National Center for Farmworker Health

Lynch, E. W. and Hanson, M. J. (1998). *Developing cross-cultural competence: A guide for working with children and their families,* Second edition. Baltimore, MD: Paul H. Brookes.

Migrant and Seasonal Farmworker Children (1998). *Migration World Magazine, 26*(5), p. 36.

Mines, R., Mullenax, N., and Saca, L. (2001). *The binational farmworker health survey: An in-depth study of agricultural worker health in Mexico and the United States.* Davis, CA: California Institute for Rural Studies.

National Center for Farmworker Health (NCFH) (2001). Migrant Health Issues: Monograph Series. Monographs 1-10. Buda, TX: Author.

National Center for Farmworker Health (NCFH) (2002). *Facts about farmworkers.* Available online at <www.ncfh.org/docs/fs-Facts%20about%20Farmworkers. pdf>.

National Research Council and Institute of Medicine (1998). *Protecting youth at work: Health, safety, and development of working children and adolescents in the United States.* Washington, DC: National Academy Press. Cited in Human Rights Watch (HRW) (2000). *Fingers to the bone: United States failure to protect child farmworkers.* New York: Author.

National Safety Council (NSC) (1989). *Accident facts.* Chicago, IL: Author.

Organista, P. B., Organista, K. C., and Soloff, P. R. (1998). Exploring AIDS-related knowledge, attitudes, and behaviors of female Mexican migrant workers. *Health and Social Work, 23*(2), 96-103.

Pardeck, J. T. (2003). An overview of family health social work practice. In F.K.O. Yuen, G. J. Skibinski, and J. T. Pardeck (Eds.), *Family health social work practice: A knowledge and skills casebook* (pp. 3-18). Binghamton, NY: The Haworth Social Work Practice Press.

Pardeck, J. T. and Yuen, F. K. O. (1999). *Family health: A holistic approach to social work practice.* Westport, CT: Auburn House.

Perilla, J. L., Wilson, A. H., Wold, J. L., and Spencer, L. (1998). Listening to migrant Voices: Focus groups on health issues in south Georgia. *Journal of Community Health Nursing, 15,* 251-263.

Rodriquez (2001). *Domestic violence series.* Migrant Health Issues: Monograph Series No. 6. Buda, TX: National Center for Farmworker Health.

Rothenberg, D. (1998). *With these hands: The hidden world of migrant farmworkers today.* New York: Harcourt Brace.

United Farm Workers of America (n.d.). *The Story of Cesar Chavez.* Available online at <www.ufw.org/cestory.htm>.

U. S. General Accounting Office (1998). *Child labor in agriculture: Characteristic and legality of work* (GAO/HEHS-98-112R). Washington, DC: U.S. Government Printing Office.

Villanueva, A. L. (1994). My people are the color of the earth. In M. M. Gillan and J. Gillan (Eds.), *Unsettling America: An anthology of contemporary multicultural poetry* (pp. 314-316). New York: Penguin.

Villarejo, D. and Baron, S. L. (1999). The occupational health and safety status of hired farmworkers. State of the art reviews. *Occupational Medicine, 14*(3), 613-635.

Villarejo, D., Lighthall, D., Williams, D. III, Souter, A., Mines, R., Bade, B., Samuels, S., and McCurdy, S. A. (2000). *Suffering in silence: A report on the health of California's agricultural workers.* Woodland Hills, CA: The California Endowment.

Von Essen, S. and McCurdy, S. A. (1998). Health and safety risks in production agriculture. *Western Journal of Medicine, 169,* 214-220.

Wilk, V. A. (1993). Health hazard to children in agriculture. *American Journal of Industrial Medicine, 24,* 283-290.

Yuen, F. K. O. (2003). Critical concerns for family health practice. In F. K. O. Yuen, G. J. Skibinski, and J. T. Pardeck (Eds.), *Family health social work practice: A knowledge and skills casebook* (pp. 19-39). Binghamton, NY: The Haworth Social Work Practice Press.

Yuen, F. K. O., Skibinski, G. J., and Pardeck, J. T. (Eds.) (2003). *Family health social work practice: A knowledge and skills casebook.* Binghamton, NY: The Haworth Social Work Practice Press.

SECTION II:
POLICY, PROGRAMS,
AND EMERGING FAMILIES

Chapter 8

Grandparents As Parents:
An Emerging Family Pattern

Christine A. Price

INTRODUCTION

The likelihood of becoming a grandparent has increased dramatically as a result of demographic changes in fertility and mortality (Pruchno and Johnson, 2000). Currently, 94 percent of older adults will experience grandparenthood, and nearly 50 percent will become great-grandparents (Hooyman and Kiyak, 1996). A direct result of the commonality of this family role has been an expanded empirical interest in the symbolic roles and functional responsibilities associated with grandparenthood.

Historically, society has viewed grandparents as peripheral to the nuclear family system, and as providers of supplemental support to parents. Common descriptions of grandparent-grandchild relationships, for example, have included grandparents serving as family historians, playmates, or as mentors to grandchildren (Kornhaber, 1996). During the 1990s a new dimension of grandparenthood emerged: the role of the custodial caregiver and surrogate parent. This newly defined grandparent role has contributed to an emerging family form, frequently referred to as the "skipped-generation" family. In these families, a grandparent, usually a grandmother, takes complete parental responsibility for raising one or more of the grandchildren. The dramatic growth in skipped generation families has altered stereotypical assumptions and expectations about what grandparenthood entails.

From 1980 to 1990 there was a 44 percent increase in the number of children living with either grandparents or relatives other than parents (Glass and Huneycutt, 2002). By 1995, according to the U.S. Census, nearly 4 million children under the age of eighteen lived in a grandparent-headed household. More specifically, 1.5 million lived in a household in which no parent was present (Hayslip et al., 2002; Poe, 2002). An estimated 50 percent of grandparents raising grand-children do so in their home with the children's mother present, whereas 1 million custodial grandparents provide care with no parent present (Glass and Huneycutt, 2002). For the purposes of this chapter, discussion will be limited to grandparent-headed households in which the grandparent is the primary provider and the adult child/parent may or may not be involved in the care of the child(ren).

According to data from the National Survey of Families and Households (NSFH), grandparent caregiving was established as a growing phenomenon that cut across racial and class lines (Fuller-Thompson, Minkler, and Driver, 2000). By using a nationally representative sample of 173 caregiving grandparents, Fuller-Thompson and associates (2000) were able to create a profile of grandparent caregivers by identifying demographic details of this population. For example, 54 percent of custodial grandparents in their sample were married, a majority were women (77 percent), and all racial/ethnic groups were represented: white (62 percent), African American (27 percent), Hispanic (10 percent), and other (1 percent). Other researchers have also found the prevalence of grandparent-headed households is disproportionate among racial groups. For example, among African-American children, 13.5 percent are likely to be raised in a grandparent-headed household compared to 6.5 percent of Hispanic children and 4.1 percent of white children (Cox, 2000). Finally, the 75 percent of custodial grandparents who take responsibility for grandchildren under the age of five and provide care for a minimum of three years illustrate the commitment and endurance associated with this role (Fuller-Thompson, Minkler, and Driver, 2000).

Researchers have consistently found grandmothers to be the primary caretakers of grandchildren in comparison to grandfathers. Although grandfather-only families are growing (Glass and Huneycutt, 2002), they are still outnumbered by grandmother-only families. In 1997, among the 4.7 million grandparents living with grandchildren, 2.9 million were grandmothers as compared to 1.7 million grand-fathers (Bryson and Casper, 1999). Coresident grandmothers frequently outnumber grandfathers for several reasons, including the higher mortality rates of men, the likelihood of older women to be widowed and to never remarry, and the assumed caregiving responsibilities of women.

Unfortunately, caregiving grandparents, especially grandmothers, frequently encounter financial hardships. In fact, custodial grandparents are 60 percent more likely than noncustodial grandparents to be living on incomes below the poverty line. The three family types most at risk for living in poverty are grandmother-headed households with a parent present, without a parent present, and single-parent households with a grandmother present (Bryson and Casper, 1999). It is important to note that in each of these family types a grandfather or father is absent. Because men are more likely to be in the labor force and frequently earn more than women, skipped-generation families without a male present are at greater risk of being financially disadvantaged.

A variety of social and cultural factors have contributed to the expansion of skipped-generation households in the United States. Included among these factors is the dramatic increase in drug and alcohol abuse witnessed during the 1980s and 1990s, increased divorce and teen pregnancy rates, the death of parents due to violence or AIDS, and stiffer judicial sentencing resulting in greater numbers of incarcerated women (Cox, 2000; Fuller-Thompson and Minkler, 2000).

CONCERNS OF CUSTODIAL GRANDPARENTS

To utilize the strengths and address the needs of custodial grandparents, it is important that researchers, policymakers, and clinicians understand the primary concerns of this population. Included among these concerns are three well-documented issues: (1) health-related problems of the custodial grandparent, (2) issues of financial insecurity, and (3) challenges associated with pursuing custody or establishing legal authority.

With regard to the health concerns of custodial grandparents, research has shown high rates of depression, poor self-rated health, and the likelihood of dealing with multiple chronic health conditions (Fuller-Thompson and Minkler, 2000). Additional studies have shown insomnia, hypertension, and back and stomach problems as concerns

(Marx and Solomon, 2000). Although the health of custodial grand-parents is generally worse than noncustodial grandparents, research-ers have found some variation based on marital status. A study by Marx and Solomon (2000) examined the health status of women liv-ing in custodial and noncustodial households. Married women who were not raising grandchildren were the healthiest, and single custo-dial grandmothers were the most disadvantaged. Compared to mar-ried custodial grandmothers, women raising grandchildren alone re-ported more chronic health problems and felt their lifestyles were severely limited due to health-related impairments. Although increas-ing age is frequently cited as the cause of increased health problems among custodial grandparents, it is important to recognize that other factors such as income and access to healthcare, the number of grand-children, and the health and behavioral characteristics of grandchil-dren can also impact the physical health of custodial grandparents. Undoubtedly, caregiving grandparents who have existing health prob-lems when they take on the responsibilities of raising grandchildren are disadvantaged and should be monitored closely. At the same time, however, grandparents with minimal health limitations are at risk of developing health complications as a result of the stressors associated with this late-life parenting role.

In addition to coping with health-related challenges, providing for grandchildren while living on a limited income is frequently cited as a primary concern of custodial grandparents. As mentioned previously, a disproportionately high percentage of caregiving grandparents live on incomes below or near poverty. Skipped-generation households are almost twice as likely to report receiving public assistance or welfare benefits (Fuller-Thompson and Minkler, 2000). Frequently, a grand-parent who takes responsibility for one or more grandchildren must continue working or return to work despite health limitations or plans to enjoy retirement. It is common for retirement funds and lifetime savings accounts to be depleted in order to provide for grandchildren. As a result, the costs associated with the surrogate-parenting role can often place the future financial security of caregiving grandparents in jeopardy.

The enactment of the Personal Responsibility and Work Opportu-nity Reconciliation Act of 1996 (PRWORA), often referred to as "welfare reform," did little to improve the financial situation of caregiving grandparents. Because the purpose of this legislation was to address problems associated with children being raised by single mothers, the PRA does not provide effective assistance to children being raised by grandparents (Mullen, 2000). When Temporary Assistance for Needy Families (TANF) replaced the long-established Aid to Families with Dependent Children (AFDC), a primary source of cash assistance for custodial grandparents ceased to exist. Because TANF is a need-based program, only families with limited incomes and resources qualify for assistance. As a result, a number of custodial grandparents may not have enough income to make ends meet but have too much income to qualify for TANF. For example, a grandparent may have an income of only $900 a month and have $1,500 in savings, yet still exceed state eligibility standards (Mullen, 2000). Although caregiving grandparents do not have to obtain legal custody to qualify for benefits, they do have to prove that the grandchild is being deprived of parental support; that they, the grandparents, are the primary caretakers of the child; and that the grandchild is residing in their home. Critics of the TANF legislation point to a number of problematic components for custodial grandparents, for example, a five-year cap on benefits, work requirements, imposed federal guidelines, and the ending of entitlement assistance (Mullen, 2000).

Beyond issues of health and financial security, custodial grandparents frequently encounter varying legal challenges associated with their caregiving role. For example, in order to provide care on a daily basis, it is critical that custodial grandparents are able to make decisions on behalf of a grandchild, access school or medical records, and/or provide consent for medical treatment (Albert, 2000). Parents may delegate this authority to a grandparent or other individual, but in cases in which parents are unable or unwilling to do so, custodial grandparents must pursue this authority through other means. A small number of states are adopting consent legislation that is informal but still provides custodial grandparents with the necessary power to make decisions. Consent legislation allows a parent to grant another individual the authority to make decisions on behalf of a child for a specific period of time or until this right is terminated by the parent. Usually the decision-making authority is limited to specific issues, such as school enrollment or medical care (Perez-Porter and Flynt, 2000). The value of this type of legislation is that the consent can be granted without going to court. More formal methods of obtaining legal authority are also available to caregiving grandparents, for example, pursuing custody of a grandchild or being awarded guardianship. Obtaining custody requires a caregiving grandparent to file a formal petition in court, and the biological parent of the child must be found unfit (Albert, 2000). Alternatively, guardianship involves the suspension of parental rights rather than complete termination. A guardian has full legal authority for a child, but the scope of this authority may depend on the type of guardianship awarded, which varies by state (Perez-Porter and Flynt, 2000). Because state legislation differs on the methods for obtaining legal authority, it is important that custodial grandparents educate themselves on the options available to them.

FAMILY HEALTH PRACTICE CONCERNS

Because the primary purpose of the family health practice approach is to achieve holistic wellness within a family system, it is critical that intervention approaches recognize the context in which families function in addition to individual development, family/group dynamics, and issues of diversity (Yuen, 2003). As previously mentioned, researchers have identified three primary concerns of custodial grandparents; these include functioning health status, issues of financial security, and difficulties in obtaining legal authority. Family practitioners who are working with caregiving grandparents must design and implement their intervention approach within the context of these existing challenges.

This chapter presents and discusses four family health practice considerations: (1) psychosocial challenges of custodial grandparents, (2) racial/ethnic considerations, (3) problem behaviors of grandchildren, and (4) negotiating relationships with adult children.

Psychosocial Challenges of Custodial Grandparents

The first of these considerations pertains to the psychosocial and emotional challenges experienced by custodial grandparents. As a direct result of their adjustment to and ongoing management of this parenting role, grandparents frequently experience a variety of conflicting emotions. For example, although custodial grandparents may feel emotional fulfillment from caregiving, they may also experience feelings of resentment at the loss of their personal freedom and shame at what they frequently view as their own parenting failure. Feelings of deprivation are a common reaction to the responsibilities of custodial grandparenting (Glass and Huneycutt, 2002). Grandparents may be deprived not only of pursuing retirement goals but also of sharing a conventional relationship with their adult child and their grandchild(ren). Unlike their peers who may spend weekends entertaining and spoiling grandchildren, these grandparents must sacrifice their dreams of traditional grandparenting and replace them with the reality of being full-time providers. Custodial grandparents also report a sense of social alienation as a result of their caregiving role (Fuller-Thompson and Minkler, 2000). Decreased social interaction with family and friends, combined with a lack of identification with persons their own age as well as other parents in school and community settings, frequently contribute to feelings of loneliness and isolation.

Caregiving grandparents often blame themselves for the actions of their adult children. As a result, they report feelings of inadequacy and doubt when faced with the task of parenting their grandchildren and being responsible for their futures. Unquestionably, the responsibilities of raising a child in the twenty-first century are dramatically different than the experience of parenting children a generation or two ago. Common worries about gangs, drugs, violence, and an openly sexual society permeate the minds of custodial grandparents. Although few educational programs specifically target this population (Chenoweth, 2000), parent education can benefit caregiving grandparents by focusing on their strengths and providing them with new tools and strategies for approaching parenthood the second time around.

Although the emotions of resentment, uncertainty, and even shame are to be expected, many grandparents feel guilty or disloyal and fear criticism for expressing any dissatisfaction or frustration with their caregiving responsibilities. Fortunately, the emergence of grandparent-caregiver support groups in all fifty states may help to address feelings of alienation and provide a safe environment for grandparents to share experiences and emotions. Because the effectiveness of these group interventions has not been documented, their potential for benefiting custodial grandparents needs further examination (Fuller-Thompson and Minkler, 2000).

Racial/Ethnic Considerations

Although a majority of custodial grandparents are white, non-Hispanic, there is a disproportionate representation of grandparents raising grandchildren among African-American and Hispanic populations (Cox, 2000; Fuller-Thompson and Minkler, 2002).

Although custodial grandparenting crosses racial boundaries, very few researchers have explored the similarities and differences between different racial/ethnic groups. A majority of the research conducted with African-American custodial grandparents has focused on those who have taken responsibility for their grandchildren as a result of the drug addiction of their adult child (Baird, John, and Hayslip, 2000). Although surrogate parenting has been a well- established pattern in the African-American community, the recent increase in the numbers of parenting grandparents has resulted in these families receiving greater attention. Circumstances surrounding custodial responsibilities and the resources available to African-American grandparents differ from their white, non-Hispanic counterparts. The limited research on African-American grandparents indicates that they are more likely to live in poverty, be forced to work past retirement age; have less education, fewer work skills, and poorer health status; and experience more physical disability in later life than whites (Brown and Mars, 2000). Studies exploring the experiences of African-American caregiving grandmothers report that custodial responsibilities do negatively impact the psychological, physical, and emotional health of this population, yet these challenges do not prevent or discourage them from providing care (Minkler, Roe, and Price, 1992). An important coping strategy implemented by these caregiving grandmothers is the frequent utilization of informal support from family, community, and religious sources.

Although custodial grandparenting is not as prevalent among Hispanic families as in African-American communities, their numbers are increasing (Cox, Brooks, and Valcarcel, 2000). Similar to African-American grandparents, Hispanic grandparents are likely to live in poverty, experience poor health and disability, and have less education. These challenges are exacerbated by their low proficiency in English and worry about immigration status and/or eligibility for public services (Cox, Brooks, and Valcarcel, 2000). Because Latino culture places a strong emphasis on the needs of the family over the individual, and the role of mother is central to the identities of women, grandmothers frequently assist their adult children in raising grandchildren. Research shows that reasons why Hispanic grandparents, usually grandmothers, assume full parental responsibilities for grandchildren are similar to those of African-American caregiving grandparents: drug addiction, HIV/AIDS, and incarceration (Cox, Brooks, and Valcarcel, 2000). Preliminary investigations of this population have revealed the experiences of Hispanic grandparent caregivers to be significantly influenced by issues of family loyalty, language barriers, access to social services, and challenges of cultural adjustment. Furthermore, census data have shown that kinship caregivers among Hispanic households are just as likely to be aunts, cousins, or godparents as they are to be grandparents (Fuller-Thompson and Minkler, 2000).

Possibly as a result of their lesser numbers, information on Native American or Asian Pacific Islander skipped-generation families is relatively nonexistent. To provide clinical support and effective interventions, it is imperative that practitioners give appropriate attention to the sociocultural variations that exist among these minority populations as well.

Problem Behaviors of Grandchildren

Many custodial grandparents are faced with raising grandchildren who display challenging emotional and/or behavioral problems (Hayslip et al., 2000). It is difficult to ascertain, however, whether these problems stem from previous time spent with a biological parent, the transition to being cared for by a grandparent, a troublesome relationship between a parent and grandparent, or a combination of these or other factors. Regardless of the cause, the high incidence of poverty, drug abuse, and neglect experienced by children in grandparent-headed homes is thought to result in an increased risk of custodial grandparents parenting a child with problems. At the same time, however, little research has been conducted on the prevalence of mental health problems among children being raised by grandparents (Hayslip et al., 2000).

Among children and adolescents in general, 14 to 22 percent exhibit some form of emotional or behavioral dysfunction during childhood or adolescence (Silverthorn and Durant, 2000). These problem behaviors are frequently classified into two categories: (1) *externalizing behaviors* that include disruptive, hyperactive, aggressive, and delinquent activities and (2) *internalizing behaviors* that refer to displays of social anxiety, depression, and withdrawal (Hayslip et al., 2000). Because externalizing behaviors are often disruptive, they are more likely to get the attention of grandparents and result in requests for assistance from mental health professionals. Unfortunately, internalizing behaviors may be more frequently overlooked or dismissed as part of the adjustment process and, as a result, intervention does not take place.

Because it is important to respond to problem behaviors early in hopes of avoiding future antisocial activity, custodial grandparents need to (1) be aware of any emotional or behavioral problems displayed by their grandchildren, (2) be open to having a mental health assessment conducted, and (3) be informed about the treatments and other psychological services available to the children in their care. Although preliminary studies indicate custodial grandparents are seeking help from school psychologists and other counseling professionals for their grandchildren with problem behaviors, there is no solid documentation pertaining to the frequency with which grandparents seek this assistance, or the effectiveness of these treatment interventions in this particular family setting (Silverthorn and Durant, 2000).

Relationships with Adult Children

A final family practice consideration is the relationship between the caregiving grandparent(s) and the adult child/parent. First, because grandparents sometimes assume parenting responsibilities as a result of death, incarceration, or abandonment, there may not be an adult child present. In these cases, the grandparent is entirely responsible for the grandchild, and no negotiation with an adult child is required. In other cases, however, in which an adult child is unable to provide care due to substance abuse, neglect, or because he or she is financially incapable, grandparents must maintain an ongoing relationship with the adult child/parent.

A frequent complaint among caregiving grandparents is the experience of relationship difficulties with the adult child/parent (Cox, 2000). For example, in families in which parental visitation has been awarded, grandparents must manage the various challenges associated with those visits. First, they must negotiate relationship boundaries with the adult child in relation to their own parent-child history as well as their current parenting of their grandchild. Second, it is often necessary to regain authority and reestablish stability and structure with grandchildren following each visit. Understandably, grandchildren may experience divided loyalties between their parents and grandparent(s), feel confused about how their parent is acting, or feel angry when the parent leaves. This may result in displays of problem behavior or emotional withdrawal on the part of the grandchild (Glass and Huneycutt, 2002). In addition, in cases of drug or alcohol abuse, parental visits may become troublesome when a grandparent is dealing with an intoxicated or otherwise impaired adult child. Grandparents who are forced to report the adult child/parent's behavior to probation officers or other legal authorities often do so with conflicted feelings of shame, anger, and exasperation, as well as concern for their child's well-being.

In skipped-generation families in which the adult child/parent lives in the grandparent-headed household, varying dynamics may apply. For some, the adult child/parent may be involved in the care of the children but not serve as the primary caregiver. Alternatively, the adult child may be an inconsistent presence that takes on no parental responsibilities with regard to their children. In many cases the grandparent and adult child negotiate their individual roles and associated responsibilities with no confusion or conflict. In other cases, however, a continuing struggle to establish and maintain clearly defined roles takes place. In families in which the parent is opposed to the grandparent providing care, or when parents and grandparents cannot agree on who provides care or how it should be provided, conflict often results (Cox, 2000). Unfortunately, whether or not this conflict takes place in front of the children, it can be emotionally and psychologically damaging to them. It is critical in these multigenerational households that parents and grandparents practice and maintain a supportive relationship that involves open communication and respect.

In the context of family health intervention, it is critical to incorporate various theoretical and developmental approaches (e.g., systems theory, developmental theories, and social constructivism). In doing so, however, it is important to be cognizant of the day-to-day reality of custodial grandparents and to assist them in identifying their strengths as well as the areas in which they need assistance. In addition to the family practice considerations already presented, custodial grandparents may also require support in managing the following needs:

1. To establish boundaries and negotiate healthy interactions with adult children
2. To seek out parent-education programs and incorporate updated parenting techniques into their interactions with grandchildren
3. To educate themselves about and respond appropriately to the changing developmental needs of grandchildren
4. To find alternative care arrangements for grandchildren should they become disabled or die
5. To locate and utilize formal and informal social support resources
6. To arrange time for themselves and attempt to preserve normative relationships with spouse, family, and friends

CONCLUSION

The number of grandparents taking full or partial responsibility for the care of their grandchildren has increased dramatically in the past two decades (Fuller-Thompson and Minkler, 2000). This shift in the conventional portrayal of grandparenthood has resulted in a growing interest among researchers, clinicians, and policymakers to document and understand the experiences of this population. Although the challenges faced by custodial grandparents are frequently emphasized and continue to be explored, the positive aspects of this emerging family form must also be recognized. Despite experiencing health limitations, financial insecurity, and ambiguous legal authority, caregiving grandparents are grateful for the close emotional bonds they establish with their grandchildren and report feelings of pleasure and relief at their ability to provide the care their grandchildren needed (Fuller-Thompson and Minkler, 2000). In addition, grandparents often experience an enhanced sense of purpose and meaning of life, and describe the fun and spontaneity their grandchildren provide.

In response to the growth of skipped-generation families, many progressive steps have taken place. Support groups have been established in all fifty states, policies advocating for the rights of custodial grandparents have been put into practice, resource centers have been developed, professional and political conferences have been designated to the needs of this population, and researchers have conducted numerous empirical studies. Despite this progress, however, considerable work has yet to be accomplished. Additional research that explores more fully the cross-racial, cross-cultural, and cross-class experiences of custodial grandparents is necessary. The identification of state and federal forms of financial assistance for caregiving grandparents remains a critical need. Finally, intervention programs that help caregiving grandparents manage and cope with their parenting responsibilities must be created, practiced, and evaluated for this particular population.

Case Study #1

Frank and Alice Matthews are a white, married couple in their sixties who are raising their three grandchildren: Daniel (age eight), Adam (age five), and Grace (age three). Their son, Neil, who is the father of the children, is a divorced, recovering drug addict. Neil has full custody of the children but is unable to provide a stable, safe home environment. In addition to his addictions, Neil has a learning disability that makes it difficult to keep a job. The children's mother, a practicing drug addict, deserted them following an ugly divorce. Although Frank and Alice do not have custody of the children, Neil has agreed to appoint them as legal guardians, which enables them to make all of the necessary decisions related to the children's care as well as apply for financial assistance.

Despite the limited financial assistance they receive on behalf of the children through TANF, Frank has been forced to return to work after having been retired for four years. Their retirement plans for traveling and Alice's hope of pursuing her talent in watercolor painting have been set aside. The Matthews feel very fortunate to have a strong marriage and rely considerably on each other, their faith, and their church community for emotional support. The issues that are troubling Frank and Alice are related to their conflicted relationship with their son and the effect of this unstable relationship on the grandchildren. Although Neil has undergone treatment for his drug and alcohol addictions, his sobriety is inconsistent. This results in his behavior remaining unstable and at times irrational and abusive. Although Neil's parental rights have been suspended, he has been awarded visitation by the court. The Matthews remain concerned about Neil's visits because they usually result in raised voices and abrupt departures. At times he arrives drunk and stumbling, whereas at other times he is sober, affectionate, and even charming. Frank and Alice still love their son and are not successful at setting boundaries and sticking to them. Neil frequently talks them into loaning him money or allowing him to visit, both of which they later regret.

Although Neil's visits are rare, the children consistently respond to them by acting out, crying for extended periods of time, or becoming very needy and insecure for days afterward. The children have appeared to flourish in the secure and stable environment Frank and Alice provide; however, they do still mourn the loss of their mother and display emotional and behavioral problems as a result of the neglect they experienced in their parent's care. The oldest child, Daniel, appears to be the most negatively effected by the disruption he has experienced. He has become increasingly defiant in his interactions with his grandparents as well as physically aggressive.

Intervention Design

- Seek counseling for the children to help them deal with the loss of their mother, the unstable behaviors and infrequent visits of their father, and the new relationship and home environment of their grandparents.
- Specifically, a mental health professional needs to assess Daniel to document the extent of his behavior problems and to design an immediate intervention.
- The Matthews need to learn to set boundaries to protect the children and themselves from Neil's manipulative behavior.
- The Matthews need to encourage/support Neil in entering a full-time drug and alcohol treatment program.
- The Matthews need to request assistance from the court to withdraw Neil's visitation privileges until he has established a sober and stable lifestyle.
- They should locate and participate in a grandparent-caregiver support group to enable them to learn from and interact with other grandparents in their situation. Also, these programs frequently have coinciding activities for the grandchildren to interact with each other and make friends with children in similar home settings.
- The Matthews should arrange for family members, friends, or other grandparents to provide child care to enable the Matthews to have more time to themselves and/or pursue activities they had originally planned to do (e.g., art classes, golf, or short weekend trips).

Case Study #2

Rosemarie Baker is a fifty-six-year-old African-American woman who, after raising three children of her own, is now responsible for raising two grandsons: Lamar (age three) and James (14 months). The boys are the children of her eldest daughter, who died from AIDS one year ago. Rosemarie has a good job driving a city bus, but, despite her health coverage and pension plan, the monthly income she brings in is never enough to cover the costs of the household. She is proud of having raised her children without public assistance and is unwilling to investigate what, if any, financial assistance is available to help her care for the boys. Although the court has awarded her full legal authority of her grandsons, Rosemarie has not legally adopted her grandsons because of the extensive court costs associated with those proceedings.

Rosemarie lives with the two boys in an inner-city apartment building that is surrounded by an economically declining neighborhood. When she was raising her three children, she exchanged child care with friends and neighbors in the building and never had to worry that the kids were not being looked after. Today, however, her neighbors remain behind closed doors, and the few friends that still live there are either not interested or not able to provide care. In addition to her difficulty in locating affordable child care, Rosemarie also feels isolated and exhausted much of the time. All of her energy goes into keeping her job and caring for her grandsons. Her remaining adult children are supportive of her parenting role but, due to their own family responsibilities, are unable to help her in any way. The friends she used to socialize with have little in common with her day-to-day experiences and rarely call her. This isolation and the boys being a constant reminder of her lost daughter contribute to periods of severe depression for Rosemarie. During those times she calls in sick to work and stays in bed for hours, barely responding to the boys' demands for attention. Recently, Rosemarie has experienced increasing health problems associated with having chronic hypertension and advancing arthritis. These health limitations are negatively affecting her ability to work as well as keep up with the demands of parenting two small children. Although Rosemarie adores her two grandsons and has no regrets about taking on the responsibility of raising them, she does worry a great deal about how she will continue to provide for them and for how long.

Intervention Design

- Rosemarie needs encouragement and assistance with identifying the financial assistance that is available to help her in caring for her grandsons.
- To address her periods of depression, Rosemarie needs one on one counseling. This individual attention could help her process

the loss of her daughter as well as learn coping strategies to assist her in managing the feelings of loneliness and despair she frequently experiences.

- Joining a support group for custodial grandparents could provide Rosemarie with new relationships and the opportunity to identify with other grandparents who are having similar experiences.
- Assistance with locating affordable child care would enable Rosemarie to work more consistently as well as provide her with a rare opportunity to socialize with friends or do something on her own, such as taking a walk, going to a movie, or grocery shopping.
- Attending parenting classes might provide Rosemarie with new parenting strategies related to discipline and role modeling as well as help her to identify and capitalize on her strengths and experience as a parent.
- It is important that Rosemarie receive health care treatment and ongoing supervision to address her hypertension and arthritis conditions. As a result of her role as a single caregiving grandparent as well as her health history, Rosemarie is at a significant risk of developing further health problems that may impede her ability to care for her grandsons.

DISCUSSION QUESTIONS AND RESOURCES

Discussion Questions

1. What are some of the reasons that grandparents assume full parental responsibility for their grandchildren?
2. In what ways is the experience of parenting different for custodial grandparents in comparison to biological parents?
3. Why is it important to explore the experiences of skipped-generation families from different racial/ethnic groups?
4. What are three primary challenges that many custodial grandparents encounter in caring for their grandchildren?
5. Why is it important for caregiving grandparents and adult children/parents to establish a relationship based on trust and respect?
6. How can the legal status (i.e., recognized legal authority) of a custodial grandparent affect the ability to care for a grandchild?

Recommended Readings

Billing, A., Ehrle, J., and Kortenkamp, K. (2002). Children cared for by relatives: What do we know about their well-being? In *New Federalism* (Series B, No. B-46 [May]) (pp. 1-7). Washington, DC: The Urban Institute.

Bryson, K. and Casper, L. (1999). Coresident grandparents and their grandchildren. In *Current population reports* (P23 198 [May] pp. 1-11). Washington, DC: U.S. Department of Commerce.

Cox, C. B. (2000). *Empowering grandparents raising grandchildren: A training manual for group leaders.* New York: Springer.

Cox, C. B. (Ed.) (2000). *To grandmother's house we go and stay: Perspectives on custodial grandparents.* New York: Springer.

Ehrle, J. and Geen, R. (2002). Children cared for by relatives: What services do they need? In *New Federalism* (Series B, No. B-47 [June]) (pp. 1-7). Washington, DC: The Urban Institute.

Ehrle, J., Geen, R., and Clark, R. (2001). Children cared for by relatives: Who are they and how are they faring? In *New Federalism* (Series B, No. B-28 [February]) (pp. 1-7). Washington, DC: The Urban Institute.

Hayslip, B. and Goldberg-Glen, R. (Eds.) (2000). *Grandparents raising grandchildren: Theoretical, empirical, and clinical perspectives.* New York: Springer.

Recommended Resources

AARP Grandparent Information Center
    <http://www.aarp.org/confacts/programs/gic.html>

Generations United (GU)
    <http://www.gu.org/>

REFERENCES

Albert, R. (2000). Legal issues for custodial grandparents. In B. Hayslip and R. Goldberg-Glen (Eds.), *Grandparents raising grandchildren: Theoretical, empirical, and clinical perspectives* (pp. 327-340). New York: Springer.

Baird, A., John, R., and Hayslip, B. (2000). Custodial grandparenting among African-Americans: A focus group perspective. In B. Hayslip and R. Goldberg-Glen (Eds.), *Grandparents raising grandchildren: Theoretical, empirical, and clinical perspectives* (pp. 125-144). New York: Springer.

Brown, D. R. and Mars, J. (2000). Profile of contemporary grandparenting in African-American families. In C. B. Cox (Ed.), *To Grandmother's house we go and stay: Perspectives on custodial grandparents* (pp. 203-217). New York: Springer.

Bryson, K. and Casper, L. (1999). Coresident grandparents and grandchildren. In *Current population reports* (P23 198 [May] pp. 1-11). Washington, DC: U.S. Department of Commerce.

Chenoweth, L. (2000). Grandparent education. In B. Hayslip and R. Goldberg-Glen (Eds.), *Grandparents raising grandchildren: Theoretical, empirical, and clinical perspectives* (pp. 307-326). New York: Springer.

Cox, C. B. (2000). Why grandchildren are going to and staying at Grandmother's house and what happens when they get there. In C. B. Cox (Ed.), *To Grandmother's house we go and stay: Perspectives on custodial grandparents* (pp. 3-19). New York: Springer.

Cox, C. B., Brooks, L. R., and Valcarcel, C. (2000). Culture and caregiving: A study of Latino grandparents. In C. B. Cox (Ed.), *To Grandmother's house we go and stay: Perspectives on custodial grandparents* (pp. 218-232). New York: Springer.

Fuller-Thompson, E. and Minkler, M. (2000). American's grandparent caregivers: Who are they? In B. Hayslip and R. Goldberg-Glen (Eds.), *Grandparents raising grandchildren: Theoretical, empirical, and clinical perspectives* (pp. 3-21). New York: Springer.

Fuller-Thompson, E., Minkler, M., and Driver, D. (2000). A profile of grandparents raising grandchildren in the United States. In C. B. Cox (Ed.), *To Grandmother's house we go and stay: Perspectives on custodial grandparents* (pp. 20-33). New York: Springer.

Glass, J. C. and Huneycutt, T. L. (2002). Grandparents parenting grandchildren: Extent of situation, issues involved, and educational implications. *Educational Gerontology, 28,* 139-161.

Hayslip, B., Emick, M. A., Henderson, C. E., and Elias, K. (2002). Temporal variations in the experience of custodial grandparenting: A short-term longitudinal study. *Journal of Applied Gerontology, 21*(2), 139-156.

Hayslip, B., Silverthorn, P., Shore, R. J., and Henderson, C. E. (2000). Determinants of custodial grandparents' perceptions of problem behavior in their grandchildren. In B. Hayslip and R. Goldberg-Glen (Eds.), *Grandparents raising grandchildren: Theoretical, empirical, and clinical perspectives* (pp. 255-268). New York: Springer.

Hooyman, N. and Kiyak, H. A. (1996). *Social gerontology: A multidisciplinary perspective,* Fourth edition. Boston: Allyn & Bacon.

Kornhaber, A. (1996). *Contemporary grandparenting.* Thousand Oaks, CA: Sage.

Marx, J. and Solomon, J. C. (2000). Physical health of custodial grandparents. In C. B. Cox (Ed.), *To Grandmother's house we go and stay: Perspectives on custodial grandparents* (pp. 37-55). New York: Springer.

Minkler, M., Roe, K., and Price, M. (1992). The physical and emotional health of grandmothers raising grandchildren in the crack cocaine epidemic. *The Gerontologist, 32,* 752-761.

Mullen, F. (2000). Grandparent and welfare reform. In C. B. Cox (Ed.), *To Grand-mother's house we go and stay: Perspectives on custodial grandparents* (pp. 113-131). New York: Springer.

Perez-Porter, M. and Flynt, M. M. (2000). Grandparent caregiving: Legal status issues and state policy. In C. B. Cox (Ed.), *To Grandmother's house we go and stay: Perspectives on custodial grandparents* (pp. 132-148). New York: Springer.

Pruchno, R. A. and Johnson, K. W. (2000). Research on grandparenting. In E. W. Markson and L. A. Hollis-Sawyer (Eds.), *Intersections of aging: Readings in social gerontology* (pp. 300-307). Los Angeles, CA: Roxbury.

Silverthorn, P. and Durant, S. L. (2000). Custodial grandparenting of the difficult child: Learning from the parenting literature. In B. Hayslip and R. Goldberg-Glen (Eds.), *Grandparents raising grandchildren: Theoretical, empirical, and clinical perspectives* (pp. 47-64). New York: Springer.

Yuen, F. K. O. (2003). Critical concerns for family health practice. In F. Yuen, G. Skibinski, and J. Pardeck (Eds.), *Family health social work practice: A knowledge and skills casebook* (pp. 19-40). Binghamton, NY: The Haworth Press.

Chapter 9

Lesbian and Gay Families: The Changing and Unsteady Legal and Social Environment

Robin Kennedy

We come from the same place. Gay or straight, this whole issue of sexuality is about two people who see each other, and just like everyone else, get a crush, have a glint in the eye, want to go out on a date, want to hold hands, want to kiss, hope that the other likes them, hope they think they're attractive. There's nothing that goes on between a gay couple that doesn't go on between a heterosexual couple.

Kathy Najimy, Actress (HRC, 2001)

INTRODUCTION

Gay and lesbian couples share the same concerns regarding parenthood that their straight counterparts face. The self-doubts and questions are the same. How will this child change our lives? What will a child do to our couple relationship? Can we afford a child? Will I be a good parent? Lesbian and gay parents face additional questions and doubts: How do we want to go about having a child? Can we afford sperm donation or a surrogate? How do we choose a sperm donor or surrogate? How can we find an accepting adoption agency? (Perrin, 2002). Is it fair to raise a child in a same-sex household when the world is still a homophobic and heterosexist place? The questions and the doubts are daunting. However, gays and lesbians are increasingly making the decision to raise children, either through adoption, insemination, or surrogacy.

Currently, the majority of children being raised in gay and lesbian households were conceived in a heterosexual relationship (Perrin, 2000). Until recently it was common for gay and lesbian individuals to lose custody of their children to their former spouse because of their sexual orientation. Although no longer the norm, a judge can still remove a child from a biological parent if he or she deems that the child "witnessing" a parent's homosexual lifestyle is "not in the best interest of the child." As Huff (2001) points out, child custody battles are some of the most emotion-laden cases brought into a courtroom. Consequently, custody cases can elicit more "emotional baggage" from a judge than almost any other type of case. Judicial bias was never more apparent than in the now famous *In re: Ward* case in Florida. A lesbian mother lost custody of her youngest daughter based solely on her sexual orientation. The court awarded custody of the child to her father, who was recently released from prison for murdering his former wife. The judge justified his actions by pointing out that the mother's older daughter was an out lesbian, and giving custody of the younger sibling to the father would "give *this* child a chance" (Custody and Visitation, 1997, p. 15).

In addition to the belief that lesbians raise lesbians (proven repeatedly to be untrue; see Patterson, 1992), judges often deny custody to a gay or lesbian biological parent due to risk of harm to the child from the social stigma attached to homosexuality. In other words, custody would be denied to a loving biological parent because we live in a homophobic society. This position is in direct violation of the Supreme Court ruling in *Palmore v. Sidoti* (1984). This was a custody case in which the white father was seeking custody of his white daughter from his ex-wife on the grounds that her new husband was African American. The father's position was that his daughter would be stigmatized and discriminated against by the racial prejudice she would have to face living in an interracial family. The Supreme Court found in favor of the mother. Justice Warren Earl Burger wrote poignantly in the ruling:

> The question is whether the reality of the private biases and the injury they might inflict are permissible considerations for the removal of an infant child from the custody of its natural mother. We have little difficulty concluding that they are not. The Constitution cannot control such prejudice but neither can it tolerate

them. Private biases may be outside the reach of the law, but the law cannot, directly or indirectly, give them effect. (*Palmore v. Sidoti,* 1984)

The lives of homosexual individuals are still today commonly filled with discrimination. Gay and lesbian families do not have the same legal rights granted to straight families. This lack of legal protection affects gay and lesbian families on a daily basis in ways that most straight families could not imagine. At the heart of this inequity is the definition of the word *family* within a legal framework. The word *family* appears 2,086 times in the U.S. Code and 4,149 times in California statutes (Robson, 1994). *Family* is rarely defined within the context of the law. The default definition is often interpreted as a close blood relation or legal commitment, such as marriage or adoption.

LEGAL INEQUITIES

Hartman (1999) has written extensively on gay and lesbian public policy, stating, "If an intimate human group is not defined as family, it is excluded from the rights, benefits, protections, and entitlements encoded in these enactments" (p. 108). Due to these inequities, lesbian and gay families are virtually invisible in the eyes of the law. The inequities span the family life cycle, from the physical act of lovemaking, to having and raising a child, to issues related to death and the distribution of property. The following sections discuss partial list of laws, policies, and benefit restrictions that affect the lives of gay and lesbian families.

Sodomy

Sodomy laws date back to King Henry VIII and have always been vague in exactly what constituted sodomy. During the nineteenth century, Pennsylvania, as well as a number of other states, started including oral sex in their sodomy laws. Some states stipulated sexual acts covered by the sodomy law were illegal for same-sex couples only. Since the 1950s, sodomy laws have been recognized as an infringement on civil rights, and most states have abolished the laws. Some of these laws have been eradicated by legislative action, and others were removed from the books by court action finding the laws unconstitutional (Eskridge, 1999). Until 2003, thirteen states still had sodomy laws on the books (Human Rights Campaign Foundation [HRC], 2002b). The 2003 Supreme Court ruling (*Lawrence v. Texas* 41 S.W. 3d 349) overturned a previous decision (*Bowers v. Hardwick*, 498 U.S. 186 [1986]) banning sodomy. This ruling not only declared the Texas sodomy law unconstitutional, but all sodomy laws pertaining to private consensual sexual relations conducted in private. *Lawrence v. Texas* decriminalized homosexuality.

Adoption

Despite the assertions of the North American Council on Adoptable Children regarding the irrelevance of parental sexual orientation, numerous agencies continue to restrict adoptions to only heterosexual couples and individuals. Some states allow gay and lesbian adoptions, whereas others have passed laws expressly prohibiting such adoptions. However, even in states that allow gay couples to adopt, county and local judges can restrict this right

Second-Parent Adoption

Relatively few states have passed legislation that allows adoption of a child by a same-sex partner (HRC, 2002b). Most states currently allow only the birth parent or one adoptive parent within the homosexual couple to have legal custody of the child. Even the states that allow gay and lesbian adoption often do not allow the *couple* to adopt the child—restricting parental rights, responsibilities, and privileges to only one member of the couple—leaving the partner (coparent) with no legal connection to the child. Because of this restriction, children are denied insurance coverage by the nonadoptive/nonbiological parent's employer, denied inheritances and social security benefits if the nonadoptive/nonbiological parent dies, denied financial support and visitation by the nonadoptive/nonbiological parent in the case of a separation, and denied medical treatment if the biological/adoptive parent is not present.

Safe School Legislation

Currently seven states and the District of Columbia have legislation that protects children in school settings from discrimination and harassment based on sexual orientation and gender identity (HRC, 2002b).

Employment Discrimination

Currently no federal statute prohibits employment discrimination on the basis of sexual orientation. In 1998, President William Clinton signed an executive order prohibiting discrimination based on sexual orientation for civilian federal employees. Twelve states and the District of Columbia currently have state laws that prohibit discrimination in employment, housing, and public accommodation (HRC, 2002b).

Hate Crimes

Although hate crimes based on sexual orientation account for 11 percent (third highest category) of all reported hate crimes every year (National Coalition of Anti-Violence Programs, 1999), only twenty-seven states currently have laws against hate crimes that include sexual preference or orientation. The federal hate crimes law (18 U.S.C. Section 245) does not include sexual preference, orientation, or identity (HRC, 2002b).

Immigration of Partner

The U.S. Immigration and Nationality Act grants spouses of U.S. citizens residency and immigration rights that same-sex couples are not granted. Fifteen other countries (Austria, Belgium, Canada, Denmark, Finland, France, German, Iceland, Israel, the Netherlands, New Zealand, Norway, South Africa, Sweden, and the United Kingdom), however, grant imigrational privileges to same-sex partners of their citizens (HRC, 2002b).

Custody Laws

Due to the lack of legal protection in gay and lesbian families, laws do not dictate custody arrangements of nonbiological and nonadoptive children in the case of a break up or death of a parent. Gay and lesbian parents can be denied custody as well as visitation privileges in favor of biological or adoptive relations. Family courts are often confronted with nonbiological, nonadoptive parents trying to seek joint custody or even visitation rights after a couple breaks up. Case law is riddled with unfortunate cases of biological relatives gaining legal custody of children after a biological or adoptive parent dies, leaving both the nonadoptive, nonbiological parent as well as the child further traumatized by the death of a loved one.

Social Security

Benefits derived from Social Security are granted on the basis of marriage and biological or adoptive relationships. Due to laws prohibiting same-sex marriage and second-parent adoptions, lesbian and gay families are excluded from survivor benefits for the partner and nonbiological and nonadopted children.

Health Insurance

The right to extend health insurance coverage to a partner and children is a decision made by the employer. Today most private and public employers still limit insurance benefits to the employee, married spouse, and biological or adopted children. When employers extend benefits to domestic partners, they do not extend those benefits to nonbiological or nonadoptive children. In addition, federal tax law requires that the employee pay taxes on partner benefits. Married couples, however, do not pay taxes on spousal benefits.

Tax Laws

U.S. tax laws fail to grant same-sex couples the same tax benefits they grant to married couples, such as filing jointly, deductions for children, reduced estate taxes, combined medical and dental expenses, and exemption from paying taxes on spousal health benefits (HRC, 2002b).

Medical Leave

The Family Medical Leave Act of 1993 permits a worker up to twelve weeks of unpaid time off the job to care for an ill family member. These benefits do not extend to gay and lesbian families. Members of same-sex couples are not granted leave for a seriously ill partner, parent of a partner, or nonbiological/nonadoptive child (HRC, 2002b).

Medical Care

Gay men and lesbians are routinely denied entrance into an intensive-care unit (ICU) or emergency room where their partner is receiving treatment. Nonbiological, nonadoptive parents are not only denied visitation rights to their children in the ICU, but if they bring their children to the emergency room without the biological/adoptive parent or a medical power of attorney signed by the biological/adoptive parent, the hospital can deny emergency treatment until the biological/adoptive parent has given permission to treat the child.

Estate Planning

In the case of death, the law allows for the distribution of property and assets to a wife or husband in a heterosexual union without a will. Gay and lesbian couples must have a will stating their wishes; however, these wills are more vulnerable to contest than those of heterosexual couples. Employers, the military, Social Security, or the Veterans Administration provide spousal benefits to a surviving heterosexual spouse, but this is not a possibility for a gay or lesbian family.

CURRENT STATE OF GAY AND LESBIAN FAMILIES

The previous is only a partial list of more than 1,000 federal benefits and protections that same-sex couples and families are denied due to the marriage ban (HRC, 2002b). Despite these obstacles, lesbian and gay parenting is on the rise. It has been the foregone conclusion for many years that gay men and lesbians do not have children. In fact, the term *lesbian mother,* to many, was an oxymoron. The reality is that this has never been true, and is in fact becoming increasingly invalid. Today, lesbians and gay men are adopting children (through both public and private agencies), giving birth through donor insemination and surrogacy, and becoming foster parents.

The exact number of children being raised by at least one gay parent varies according to the source. The American Civil Liberties Union (ACLU, 1999) reports the range of 6 to 14 million. According to the 2000 Census, lesbian and gay families reside in 99.3 percent of all the counties in the United States, with a total of 601,209 gay and lesbians families reported (HRC, 2001). Although this represents a dramatic increase in same-sex couples since the 1990 Census, fear of discrimination leads one to believe that this number is still grossly underrepresentative of the actual numbers of same-sex families.

In researching legislative action in 2002 that affects lesbian and gay families, one is struck by the contradictions. Whereas California enacted the most comprehensive domestic partnership law to date, Michigan enacted a law that prohibits domestic-partner benefits for legislators or legislative employees. Prior to the landmark *Lawrence v. Texas* ruling, either through legislation or court action, three states (Arizona, Minnesota, and Washington) struck down sodomy laws. However, three states (Texas, Louisiana, and Montana) introduced legislation to overrule sodomy laws, which failed. Twelve states have laws prohibiting discrimination based on sexual orientation, and as well in 2002, two states expanded their nondiscriminatory legislation. However, Houston, Texas, voters approved a measure prohibiting domestic-partner benefits to municipal employees.

According to Hartman (1999, p. 93),

> This nation is going through a period of rapid social change, even a social revolution, in terms of attitudes about and policies directed at gay men and lesbians, with the result that gay people occupy what might be called a liminal position, betwixt and between acceptance and continued rejection.

These are truly strange times in which we live. Currently, eight states and 129 local governments offer benefits to the domestic partners of government employees. Maine, California, and Washington—all states that offer domestic-partnership benefits to state employees—have recently passed anti–gay marriage legislation (HRC, 2002b).

On May 17, 2004, Massachusetts began allowing same-sex marriages. Vermont offers civil unions as a substitute for marriage. This legal union allows the couple the same (state-supported) benefits and protections of marriage *only* within the state of Vermont. State-supported civil unions still have no effect on heterosexist federal regulations.

To say that all or even most of the gay population is in favor of legalizing same-sex unions would be an overstatement. There is in fact a great deal of tension within the gay and lesbian communities regarding the benefits and liabilities of marriage. To many, the institution of marriage is a formal recognition of commitment as well as protection from a homophobic society, whereas others find marriage an exclusionary, oppressive, and conservative institution created by and for a straight world. Eskridge (1996) postulates that if lesbians and gay men marry, they will become more and more like straight couples. It is this very thought that worries many in the gay and lesbian communities.

The good news is, currently, gay and lesbian families are beginning to be recognized in the work setting. Of the Fortune 500 companies, more than 200 now offer domestic-partner benefits. Apple Computer, Sun Microsystems, and Nike have offered domestic-partner benefits since 1993 and 1994. The 2002-2003 additions include Merck and Company, Proctor and Gamble, and R. J. Reynolds (HRC, 2003). The bad news is with each step forward there are antigay groups who wish to take away the legal protection gay and lesbian families have fought for. Antigay strategies often include court challenges to gay-friendly legislation, use of scare tactics intended to result in an antigay referendum ballot item, or organizing boycotts against the companies listed previously as well as all companies who recognize and support gay and lesbian families. These are the same groups that oftentimes label themselves "pro-family." The rationale for their antigay and antifamily campaign is their rather narrow definition of family. Antigay groups often proclaim that gay and lesbian families are seeking "special privileges" and that giving gay and lesbian families the legal protections afforded heterosexual families would threaten the "traditional family." The moral high ground of antigay groups focuses on the content of the nuclear family (gender of parents, number of parents, and so on) while ignoring the quality of family relationships.

After years of psychological (American Psychological Association [APA], 1995) and sociological (Stacey and Biblarz, 2001) studies, overwhelming evidence suggests that the sexual orientation of a parent has little to do with an individual's ability to be a good parent. The American Psychological Association, the Child Welfare League of America, the North American Council on Adoptable Children, American Academy of Pediatrics, and the American Psychoanalytic Association have all issued policy statements that maintain an individual's sexual orientation is irrelevant to an individual's ability to be a good parent (HRC, 2002c). Recently, the American Academy of Pediatrics (2002, p. 339) released a statement in support of second-parent adoptions:

> Because these families and children need the permanence and security that are provided by having 2 fully sanctioned and legally defined parents, the Academy supports the legal adoption of children by coparents or second parents. Denying legal parent status through adoption to coparents or second parents prevents these children from enjoying the psychological and legal security that comes from having 2 willing, capable, and loving parents.

And Laird (1994) has noted,

> How can it be that in a world in which lesbians and gays are subjected to invisibility, silence, homophobia, and other forms of prejudice and discrimination, so many of these individuals, couples, families, and children seem to be doing as well as everyone else? . . . Could it be that lesbians and their families have special experiences and special strengths that give parents and children alike the courage to master adversity. (p. 122)

LEGAL INTERVENTIONS

A number of interventions can at least minimize the inequities that gay and lesbian families face. It is strongly recommended that gay and lesbian parents consult an attorney to discuss the documents needed in their state to protect their family. Because so many of the legal inequities can become apparent during routine medical care, medical emergencies, or death, it is the job of medical social workers to become acquainted with the legal interventions needed in their locale. Proud Parenting (2003) suggests gay and lesbian couples seek the advice of an attorney and consider the following legal documents:

1. *Will:* Details the division of property as well as guardianship of children
2. *Durable power of attorney:* Gives an individual the power to act on one's behalf in the case of incapacitation
3. *Designation of health care surrogate:* Designates an individual to make health care decisions on one's behalf should one become unable to make decisions for oneself
4. *Living will:* Otherwise known as an "advanced directive"; speaks for an individual when he or she is unable to do so, and advises health care personnel as well as the family in the individual's wishes regarding advanced life support
5. *Designation of preneed guardian:* Allows one to designate the individual chosen to be guardian in the case of incapacitation
6. *Designation of preneed guardian for minor child:* Allows one to designate a guardian for one's child in the case of incapacitation
7. *Beneficiary designations:* Makes certain all insurance policies and accounts are up to date with the desired beneficiary named
8. *Cohabitation agreement:* Written and signed by a gay or lesbian couple residing together that lays out the financial and domestic responsibilities of each partner both during the relationship and in the event of a breakup
9. *Coparenting agreement:* If one is the biological or adoptive parent of a minor child being raised in a coparenting gay relationship, a coparent agreement authorizes the nonbiological, nonadoptive parent to consent to medical care; stipulates the child's guardianship in the case of incapacitation; and stipulates each parent's rights and responsibilities in the case of a breakup

HEALTH CARE FOR GAY AND LESBIAN FAMILIES

Past research has found that gay and lesbian parents have had more positive than negative experiences with health care providers (Perrin and Kulkin, 1996). The most frequently cited positive experiences with health care providers by gay and lesbian parents included: maintaining eye contact with both parents, referring to both parents as "the parents of . . . ," and medical personnel acknowledging that the families were different and vulnerable to prejudice. One study respondent stated, "They keep trying to normalize us by saying it's just like any other family. We are not, though, and our kids will experience situations any other family will not. While differences are not necessarily deficits, we do need extra support" (Perrin and Kulkin, 1996, p. 633). In the Perrin and Kulkin (1996) research, 23 percent of the parent respondents reported they had not disclosed their sexuality to their pediatrician. One of these respondents stated, "I fear that heterosexual providers might see my son as coming from a deprived rather than different family. Sensitivity is good, but pity is misplaced" (p. 632). This research proposed three recommendations that pediatric health care providers should incorporate into their practice to encourage gay and lesbian families to disclose as well as create an overall feeling of safety:

1. Create a physical environment that welcomes diversity, that is, books, magazines, and posters that portray a number of different constellations of families.
2. Display a confidentiality statement displayed in the waiting area, assuring the patients that the staff will safeguard the family's information.
3. Make sure medical forms are not gender specific and are inclusive of gay and lesbian families.

Because the environment for gay and lesbian families can often range from tolerant to hostile, it is vital that social workers stay current on information regarding obstacles facing these unique families. Staying abreast of laws and legal interventions to assist families in negotiating the sometimes confusing and often hostile medical arena has become a vital part of practice.

Outside of social work, most health professionals get little or no training in gay and lesbian issues (Harrison, 1996). There are numerous ways to prepare oneself and one's work setting to assist gay and lesbian families:

1. Within the health care setting, take an honest inventory of individual biases regarding homosexual individuals raising chil-

dren. If biases regarding homosexual families are present, take a look at the research. Numerous studies (as well as professional organizations) attest to the fitness of gay and lesbian individuals to parent. This should take care of cognitive skepticism—and if there are still reservations, call it what it is: homophobia.

2. Examine the forms used to gather medical information. Are the forms gender neutral? Can gay and lesbian families answer the questions on the form without having to mark through hetero-sexist language?

3. Do the health care providers in the setting use gender-neutral language when getting a verbal medical history or when conversing with patients/clients?

4. Health care providers need to keep abreast of current laws affecting gay and lesbian families. Currently, these laws can both limit the rights of as well as empower gay and lesbian families.

5. Social workers, in particular, need to be kept informed of the needed legal documents that allow gay and lesbian families to operate in the most supportive and least restrictive fashion (coparent agreement, durable power of attorney, etc.). Gay advocates will often provide in-service training, free of charge, for the purposes of educating and sensitizing professional organizations to gay and lesbian issues.

THE DEVELOPMENTAL STAGES OF A GAY/LESBIAN FAMILY

The issues families face in relation to the parents' being gay change as the family evolves and as children reach developmental milestones. If peer support is available, this is helpful at all stages of individual and family development.

Preschool Years (Birth to Age Four)

The most cited challenges during the preschool period involved explaining how the child came to be in the family, that is, adoption, insemination, surrogacy, and so forth (Perrin and Kulkin, 1996). Gold and colleagues (1994) suggest this time period as an ideal time to begin this conversation with the child. As with any child at this age, do not give the child more information than she or he is requesting because it will cause confusion. Instead, focus conversations on the many different constellations of families that can exist. Engaging in conversations in which the parents and child(ren) creatively describe their own family constellation not only answers their questions but also helps prepare the child for future questions from peers (Ahmann, 1999).

School Years (Age Five to Eleven)

Children become more aware of being "different" during this time. Combined with many children's first exposure to gay jokes and generalized homophobia, it can be a particularly rough period for children of gay and lesbian parents. It is quite natural that children would try to conceal their parents' sexuality during this time. At this age children become aware of what their parents have known for quite some time: the decision to come out is a decision that is made every day, and made differently every day. Children learn when, where, and to whom they can talk with honestly about their family. It is vital that children be allowed to make their own decisions regarding to whom they give family information. The child's comfort as well as confidence depends on his or her ability to control what information is given to friends regarding their family.

Early Adolescence (Ages Twelve to Fourteen)

This stage is characterized by two prominent features: sexuality and conformity. Sexual identity and orientation become prominent during this period. At the same time, adolescents often become overly concerned with peer acceptance. Parents of children who have historically been accepting and proud of their gay heritage may feel confused or rejected by their adolescent's newly acquired embarrassment of their family (Ahmann, 1999).

Late Adolescence (Ages Fifteen to Nineteen)

This is a stage marked with conflict for all families, gay and straight. Some of the uniquely gay family difficulties center around sexuality. This is a normal time for rebellion and dissatisfaction with parents; however, in gay families, this rebellion can be directed at the parent in the form of scorning sexual orientation (Perrin and Kulkin, 1996). It is common for all adolescents to feel discomfort in bringing a date home for family introductions, and children (especially hetero-sexual children) of gay and lesbian parents may feel awkward about their family composition (Ahmann, 1999). On a positive note, re-search has shown that gay and lesbian families engage in more con-versations regarding sexuality and diversity than straight families. Consequently, these children seem to be more open and accepting of different lifestyles (Kirkpatrick, Smith, and Roy, 1981).

Case Study

Gina Sanders and Louise Wright rushed their five-year-old daughter, Katie Wright, to the emergency room at a Tampa Bay hospital. Katie had been running a fever with flulike symptoms for approximately twenty-four hours. When Tylenol failed to bring down the fever, Katie's pediatrician had advised her parents by phone to bring Katie to the emergency room of a lo-cal hospital. Katie's diagnosis eluded the usual battery of emergency room tests, and she was admitted to the pediatric unit for further observation.

Although Louise suffered from lupus, her devotion to her daughter and caring for her ill child took precedence over her own health issues. Gina took on the job of caring for Katie, Louise, and the family pets. The pace was gru-eling, but her face lit up at the sight of her daughter. Both of Katie's mothers remained at her bedside, taking turns stroking her hair, reading her stories, and singing her favorite songs, never leaving her alone. Nursing staff would often comment to Katie's parents as well among themselves how fortu-nate Katie was to have two doting mothers. One nurse commented that Katie's last name was the only way she knew who the legally recognized mother was.

Both mothers obviously shared an intimate bond with their daughter; however, only Louise could sign medical treatment consents on Katie's be-half. For this reason, Louise rarely left the hospital. Often exhausted from her own illness, Louise slept in the chair beside Katie's bed and in waiting rooms when Katie was undergoing diagnostic procedures. It was on Katie's fourth day of hospitalization that her diagnosis of a rare and chronic kidney disease was revealed. After the family had been given time to absorb the severity and duration of Katie's illness, the renal treatment team (pediatric nephro-logy specialists, MD, nurse, and social worker) met with Gina and Louise to discuss the upcoming months of treatment.

Discussion Questions

1. Looking at the list of laws and benefit restrictions mentioned earlier in the chapter, identify the most pressing problems this family faces unique to their lesbian status.
2. How can the nephrology social worker address this family in a way that both supports the family yet stays within the constraints of the law?
3. Is it important to know if Louise is the adoptive or biological mother of Katie?
4. What responsibilities does the social worker have to educate/sensitize the doctors, nursing staff, and the ancillary professionals who come in contact with this family?
5. The practitioner's relationship with this family is governed by three areas of policy: (1) the law, (2) the National Association of Social Workers (NASW) Code of Ethics, and (3) hospital policy. These three policy areas may overlap and even contradict. Identify possible scenarios in which this could be the case, then identify which policy takes precedence.

SUGGESTED READINGS

Ahmann, E. (1999). Working with families having parents who are gay or lesbian. *Pediatric Nursing, 25,* 531-536.
American Civil Liberties Union (ACLU) (1999). ACLU fact sheet: Overview of lesbian and gay parenting, adoption and foster care. Available online at: <www.aclu.org/issues/gay/parent.html>.
Benkov, L. (1994). *Reinventing the family: Lesbian and gay parents.* New York: Crown.
Human Rights Campaign Foundation (HRC). Available online at <www.hrc.org/familynet>.
Johnson, S. M. and O'Connor, E. (2001). *For lesbian parents.* New York: Guilford Press.
Laird, J. and Green, R. J. (Eds.) (1996). *Lesbians and gays in couples and families: A handbook for therapists.* San Francisco: Jossey-Bass.
Stacey, J. and Biblarz, B. J. (2001). (How) Does sexual orientation matter? *American Sociological Review, 66,* 159-183.

REFERENCES

Ahmann, E. (1999). Working with families having parents who are gay or lesbian. *Pediatric Nursing, 25,* 531-536.

American Academy of Pediatrics (2002). Coparent or second parent adoption by same-sex parents. *Pediatrics, 109,* 339-340.

American Civil Liberties Union (ACLU) (1999). ACLU fact sheet: Overview of lesbian and gay parenting, adoption and foster care. Available online at <www.aclu.org/issues/gay/parent.html>.

American Psychological Association (APA) (1995). Lesbian and gay parenting. Available online at <www.apa.org/pi/parent.html>.

Custody and visitation (1997). *Lambda Update 14*(1), 15

Eskridge, W., Jr. (1996). *The case for same-sex marriage: From sexual liberty to civilized commitment.* New York: Simon & Schuster.

Eskridge, W., Jr. (1999). *Gaylaw.* Cambridge, MA: Harvard University Press.

Gold, M. A., Perrin, E. C., Futterman, D., and Friedman, S. B. (1994). Children of gay and lesbian parents. *Pediatrics in Review, 15,* 354-358.

Harrison, A. E. (1996). Primary care of lesbian and gay patients: Educating ourselves and our students. *Family Medicine, 28*(11), 10-23.

Hartman, A. (1999). The long road to equality: Lesbians and social policy. In J. Laird (Ed.), *Lesbians and lesbian families* (pp. 91-120). New York: Columbia University Press.

Huff, E. P. (2001). The children of homosexual parents: The voices the courts have yet to hear. *American Journal of Gender, Social Policy and the Law.* Available online at <www.wcl.american.edu/journal/genderlaw/09/9-3huff.pdf>.

Human Rights Campaign Foundation (HRC) (2001). Gay and lesbian families in the United States: Same-sex unmarried partner households. Available online at <www.hrc.org/familynet/documents/l%20census.pdf>.

Human Rights Campaign Foundation (HRC) (2002a). Domestic partner benefits. Available online at <www.hrc.org/worknet/asp_search/results.asp?skey=listand list=landt=dp>.

Human Rights Campaign Foundation (HRC) (2002b). The state of the family: Laws and legislation affecting gay, lesbian, bisexual, and transgendered families. Available online at <www.hrc.org/familynet/documents/SoT.F.pdf>.

Human Rights Campaign Foundation (HRC) (2002c). What child welfare and health experts say about gay and lesbian parenting. Available online at <www.hrc.org/familynet/printpage.asp?table= chaptersandID=184>.

Human Rights Campaign Foundation (HRC) (2003). The state of the workplace 2003. Available online at: <www.hrc.org/Content/ContentGroups/Publications1/State_of_the_Workplace/SOTW_03.pdf>.

Kirkpatrick, M., Smith, C., and Roy, R. (1981). Lesbian mothers and their children: A comparative study. *American Journal of Orthopsychiatry, 51,* 545-551.

Laird, J. (1994). Lesbian families: A cultural perspective. In M. Mirkin (Ed.), *Women in context* (pp. 118-148). New York: Guilford Press.

National Coalition of Anti-Violence Programs (1999). Anti-lesbian, gay, bisexual and transgender violence in 1998 (Annual Report). New York: Author.

Palmore v. Sidoti 466 Sup. Ct. 429 (1984). Available online at: <www.caselaw. LP. findlaw.com/scripts/getcase.PL?navby=search&court=US&case=/us/466/429. html>.

Patterson, C. J. (1992). Children of lesbian and gay parents. *Child Development, 63,* 1025-1042.

Perrin, E. C. (2002). Technical report: Coparent or second parent adoption by same-sex parents. *Pediatrics, 109,* 341-344.

Perrin, E. C. and Kulkin, H. (1996). Pediatric care for children whose parents are gay or lesbian. *Pediatrics, 97,* 629-635.

Proud Parenting (2003). Protecting yourself and your family. Available online at <www.proudparenting.com/page.cfm? sectionid=118andstoryset=yes>.

Robson, R. (1994). Resisting the family: Repositioning lesbians in legal theory. *Signs, 19,* 975-996.

Stacey, J. and Biblarz, B. J. (2001). (How) Does sexual orientation matter? *American Sociological Review, 66,* 159-183.

Chapter 10

When the Family Becomes the State: Child Welfare and Foster Care Policies Affecting Family Health and Well-Being

Susan A. Taylor

INTRODUCTION

The focus of this chapter is the interface of policies and service delivery systems as they affect the health and well-being of families and children connected to the child welfare system. Because of the complexity of these features, health care professionals face unique legal, institutional, and treatment barriers in the provision of and access to quality care for this population. Understanding these complexities and their impact upon the health and well-being of this population allows health care practitioners to anticipate difficulties, develop multiple intervention paths for care delivery, and navigate competing systems of care.

To further the knowledge base needed to enhance skill development in this area, the chapter addresses the following content: (1) the nature and scope of the child welfare system and child protection policies, (2) competing and contradictory policies affecting children and families as consumers within the greater child welfare system, (3) the nature of health policy as it relates to children in out-of-home care, and (4) health-related policy and service delivery recommendations for children in out-of-home care. A case study with discussion questions has been included to provide skill building in this practice area.

THE CHILD WELFARE SYSTEM: A GRADUATED APPROACH TO STATE INTERVENTION

The child welfare system is composed of a maze of interventions based in law, governmental policies, agency formal and informal policies, interfacing and competing service delivery systems, and differing philosophies of treatment that involve "the state" in the life of the family. These policies and programs vary on a continuum of least restrictive to most restrictive, depending upon the nature of state involvement and the social, political, and economic contexts of the family in the societal milieu.

In its least restrictive form, the conglomeration of policies, programs, and interventions provide a safety net to assist vulnerable families. In its most restrictive form, the state acts as a social control agent, dictating the parameters of family and family life (Bould, 1993; Crawford, 1999; Hutchison and Charlesworth, 2000; Mason and Mauldon, 1996). The degree of state involvement in child welfare has been rationalized and sanctioned by many variables, including but not limited to economic, race, gender, sexual orientation, religion, and immigration status of parents and/or children. The lack of consistency in state involvement, however, has left a patchwork of contradictory interventions across different levels of practice (i.e., macro, mezzo, micro) and policy development (federal, state, local) through which human-service practitioners must navigate (Charlow, 2001; Downey, 2000/2001; Heck and Parker, 2002; Junek and Thompson, 1999).

From a service perspective, the child welfare system is composed of three gradations of service delivery. This continuum of services includes supportive, supplemental, and substitute services primarily directed toward low-income and low-middle-income families (Cohen, 2000; Crosson-Tower, 2001). These service groupings are not mutually exclusive. Rather, they are often used concurrently in seeking the best interest of the child within the family. This is particularly true of supportive and supplemental services used as preventive measures in reducing family stress and poverty. Understanding the graduated approach to intervention in family life is helpful for health practitioners, because the more restrictive the treatment options and service expectations, the more likely the family is participating involuntarily with the state.

CHILD WELFARE SERVICE DIFFERENTIATION

The first avenue of intervention with families and children who enter the broad service delivery system known as child welfare are services that provide social and community support to family members. Supportive services "support, reinforce, and strengthen the ability of parents and children to meet the responsibilities of their respective statuses" (Kadushin and Martin, 1988, p. 83). The purpose of these services is to provide prevention against family dissolution and child maltreatment due to social and economic factors. Often called home-based services—because they are designed to keep children at home rather than in out-of-home care—such programs include

1. school-based programs (e.g., Healthy Start, Head Start, school lunch, parenting education, informational and referral for pre-natal/postnatal care, latchkey after-school programs);
2. community health and mental health programs (e.g., providing marriage, family, and individual counseling; stress management classes and groups; and self-help groups such as Al-Anon, Alateen);
3. regional centers for developmentally challenged parents and children (e.g., providing testing, parent education and training, and mutual aid networks); and
4. community-based programs (e.g., Big Brothers Big Sisters, community athletic leagues, after-school tutoring, and General Educational Development [GED] classses).

These programs view the family holistically, recognizing the importance of social and community supports in strengthening the bonds within the family and reducing the stress of daily family life.

The second type of service intervention within the child welfare system addresses the impact of economic disparity on the lives of some families. Supplemental services include a variety of income-maintenance programs such as Temporary Assitance for Needy Families (TANF), food stamps, Women Infants and Children (WIC), Supplemental Security Income (SSI), Medicaid, workers compensation, and unemployment insurance (Cohen, 2000). These programs are income or in-kind transfer programs designed to supplement family income and provide for the health and well-being of family members.

Such programs serve the function of family preservation in addressing temporary loss of income, emotional and personal crises, child care, in-home service and treatment (e.g., home health, in-home counseling), family nutrition, mother and child nutrition, and preventive and catastrophic health care needs. If used concurrently with support services, the combined emphasis enhances family stability across multiple levels of need (economic, psychological, social) and assists families in developing and maintaining family relationships.

The third type of intervention—substitutive services—is the most restrictive in that it places the state specifically in the role and function of parent. Services included in this grouping are "temporary shelter care, foster family care, adoptive homes, group homes, residential treatment facilities, institutions" (Cohen, 2000, p. 50), kinship care, and emergency respite care (hospital-based). Generally referred to as out-of-home care, these various configurations place the child with caregivers determined suitable by the state. It is assumed that these caregivers can better provide for the safety, health, and physical well-being of the child. These interventions are mandated by the state in situations in which there is "chronic neglect and/or abuse . . . the absence of parents . . . [and/or] the child's or youth's serious emotional or behavioral problems" cannot be met within the family structure (Cohen, 2000, p. 51). It is at this level of most restrictive state intervention that the health care needs of children become complicated by the complexities inherent in institutional care. At the heart of the issue is the physical versus legal custody or guardianship of the child, and what legal limitations exist regarding who can authorize medical intervention, treatment, care, and financing. Health care decisions for these children are directly affected by this legal quagmire.

Policies of Contradictory Care

Also affecting treatment options and interventions for this population is the degree to which the multiple family-service systems do not interface (Lewandowski and GlenMaye, 2002; Kronebusch, 2001). This creates additional problems for already vulnerable families. There are many examples of this lack of collaboration, but the lack of interface between income maintenance, substance abuse, and child protective services systems is particularly poignant. Recent policy and service delivery developments in each of these areas has created a smaller funnel through which families in need can receive assistance. With changing eligibility criteria, time limitations on access of services, and restrictive reimbursement requirements on treatment these programs and program goals are often contradictory to one another in supporting the overall welfare of the family (Heck and Parker, 2002; Halfon et al., 1999). These contradictory guidelines can, in fact, put the family at greater risk of dissolution.

The interface of the Personal Responsibility and Work Opportunity Reconciliation Act and the Adoption and Safe Families Act provides a good example of the issue of contradictory policy and its impact. In 1996, the Personal Responsibility and Work Opportunity Reconciliation Act (PRWORA) (Public Law 104-193) was enacted by Congress. This act did away with AFDC (Aid to Families with Dependent Children) and replaced it with TANF (Greenberg, 2001; Hagen, 1999). The original program was designed to provide an economic floor for poor families by supplementing family income with assistance received from the government (Machtinger, 1999). The AFDC program was not time limited, and it acted as the main eligibility vehicle through which poor families became income eligible for other supplemental services (e.g., Medicaid, low-income housing, and food stamps). TANF, on the other hand, has as its primary thrust in parental work requirements, time line limitations, and requirements that adults with substance abuse problems seek treatment or lose eligibility for TANF. PRWORA also eliminated welfare as an entitlement, thereby eliminating universal eligibility. In short, simply being poor does not make one eligible for assistance from the government or private health and social welfare agencies.

On the heels of welfare reform (PRWORA) came the 1997 Adoption and Safe Families Act (ASFA) (Public Law 105-89). This act is by far the most comprehensive piece of legislation that has been enacted by Congress regarding accountability of the child welfare system for outcomes of foster placement and adoption of children under its care. One aspect of the program that has proved somewhat problematic is that it puts biological parents and children at odds within the child welfare protective services system (Stein, 2000). Unlike previous legislation that emphasized family support and preservation, this legislation focused primarily upon the welfare of the child—expediting the child's exit from foster care to availability for adoption by terminating parental rights within specified time lines

(Hutchison and Charlesworth, 2000). Specifically, under ASFA the system was required to do concurrent planning for both reunification and termination during the time the child was in out-of-home placement.

Where do the systems collide? Poverty is one of the leading indicators of child risk (health and welfare), yet the social support system (in the child welfare system denoted as supportive and supplemental) for poor families has become politically and socially unfavorable and, therefore, is diminishing (as is apparent from the enactment of PRWORA). It is anticipated that as families begin to lose their welfare benefits and lifetime eligibility the level of family poverty will increase, thereby putting children at greater risk both economically and physically from increased stress in families, which can lead to child maltreatment due to the family's inability to provide adequate health care, nutrition, housing, and education for the child. It is expected, as a result, that many of these children will enter child-protective care (foster care) (Geen and Waters, 1997). Should the parent not be able to adequately provide for the child within months, ASFA requires termination of parental rights. Also, should the parent be involved in a substance abuse treatment plan, either as one of the original terms at the time of placement in foster care or because such behavior developed during the course of the child's removal, it is unlikely that, due to the long waiting lists at substance abuse treatment programs, the parent will have received treatment and be stable prior to the time limits established in ASFA for termination of parental rights. In short, a poor parent's desire to stabilize the family's economic situation and regain physical custody of the child is largely dependent upon his or her ability to become economically stable and/or become substance free within an arbitrary time line established by law. Although states have some flexibility in the implementation of the time limit, the combination of contradictory policy objectives established in ASFA and PRWORA in essence work against the reunification of the family.

Family and Children's Health Within the Context of Child Welfare Services

Wurtele (1999) notes that research indicates, of children entering the foster care system, 53 percent enter due to neglect, 26 percent due to physical abuse, 14 percent due to sexual abuse, and 5 percent due to emotional abuse (p. 151). Although the numbers vary (Takayama, Wolfe, and Coulter, 1998; Tatara, 1993) the overriding factor in the decision for placement is the prevalence of neglect (McLoyd, 1998; Silver, 1999; Sobel, 2000). Why is this significant? Families with fewer resources in many cases have less ability to provide the necessary provisions that contribute to positive health outcomes for children. With family policy shifting away from financing for supplemental and supportive care, many families are facing a greater likelihood of the only choice being substitutive intervention.

What are the health-related issues that affect children after the state has intervened? Although scholarship clearly indicates that children who have been abused and neglected are at particularly high risk of health and mental health related problems (American Association of Pediatrics [AAP], 1997; Child Welfare League of America [CWLA], 1988; Morrison et al., 1999; Silver, Haecker, and Forkey, 1999; Szilagyi, 1998; Takayama, Wolfe, and Coulter 1998), state intervention does not always result in the timely attention to those problems (Simms et al., 1999; Sobel and Healy, 2001; U.S. General Accounting Office, 1995; Wolfe and Coulter, 1998). This is due to several factors relating to the fragmentation of policy, programmatic and financing issues across multiple care-delivery systems (Sobel and Healy, 2001; Ullman and Hill, 2001). As such, some of those issues are specific to the financing system for the delivery of health care to low-income children (Rosenbaum et al., 2001; Selden, Banthin, and Cohen, 1999; Wurtele, 1999), the child welfare system (Wulczyn and Orlebeke, 2000), and the health care delivery system as a whole (Simms et al., 1999).

The inherent policy and service issues associated with the Medicaid program (e.g., access, reimbursement rates, and types of services covered) affect this population directly (Kaiser Family Foundation, 1996; Waxman and Alker, 1996; Yudkowsky, Cartland, and Flint, 1990) since Medicaid is the primary source of funding for health and mental health services for children and adolescents in out-of-home placements (English, Morreale, Stinnett, 1999; Halfon and Berkowitz, 1993; Rosenbach, 2001). Other sources of funding such as the State Children's Health Insurance Program (SCHIP) and Title V, have helped lessen total reliance upon Medicaid as sole funder. However, funding patterns vary within states.

The reliance upon Medicaid funding creates several problems in service provision. First, there are often large gaps in time between removal of the child and when a dependency petition is filed. During that time children are in medical limbo, that is, the child may be ineligible for Medicaid. It may also be unclear as to who can give consent for medical care.

In addition, many health care providers will not accept Medicaid because of the low reimbursement rate. This also causes delays in assessment and treatment. The final issue associated with Medicaid is the limited array of services covered. Unless supplemented with other funding, children reliant only on Medicaid may have limited or no access to dental or mental-health treatment.

On a more positive note, there is policy precedent for screening and treatment. The Early and Periodic Screening, Diagnostic, and Treatment Program (EPSDT) is a federally mandated program (within Medicaid) which was developed to ensure that children in foster care "receive comprehensive well-child care, medical histories, physical exams, developmental assessments, laboratory screening, and immunizations" (Sobel and Healy, 2001, p. 496). Although many states have been lax in implementing the program requirements, that the requirements exist provides leverage for health and human service providers to create a comprehensive health agenda for this population. Identifying similar avenues of limited or unfunded policy mandates provide programmatic templates for seeking other sources of programmatic financing (Selden, Banthin, and Cohen, 1999).

Also potentially problematic in meeting the health and mental health needs of children in state custody are issues present in the child welfare system itself. First, the degree of staff turnover among child welfare employees, caseworkers, and caregivers creates a void in available consistent information concerning children in their care (Mor-Barak, Nissly, and Levin, 2001). Because of this, knowledge of health and mental health issues related to a particular child may vary as well as an understanding of the overall health and mental health needs of children entering placement. In instances in which there is high turnover of staff within the system, such measures as increased training, collaborative treatment models, and medical passports (computerized or paper) have been introduced to track the medical needs of children in state care. Although caseworkers and foster care parents are vital in collecting and maintaining medical histories on children in their care, electronic medical passports linked to the state Medicaid reimbursement system allow for fluctuations in personnel without the loss of information. In short, however, there is no consistent policy among the federal government, states, or localities as to how to address children's health issues while in state care.

WHAT CHILDREN NEED

Templates related to the health care needs of children in out-of-home placements have been developed by major child advocacy groups in the past fifteen years. Most recently, the Committee on Early Childhood Adoption and Dependent Care, of the American Academy of Pediatrics (AAP) (2002), published several recommendations related to meeting the health and mental health needs of children in out-of-home care. These recommendations built on the 1988 suggestions made by the Child Welfare League of America (CWLA). The CWLA's proposed guidelines were developed in conjunction with the AAP.

Special consideration was also given by the Committee on Early Childhood Adoption and Dependent Care to recommendations made in 2001 by District II of the American Academy of Pediatrics' Task Force on Health Care for Children in Foster Care. Combined, these recommendations led the committee to suggest the following guidelines:

1. Pediatricians should participate in the care of children in foster care as primary care physicians and as consultants to child welfare agencies. Child welfare agencies, general pediatricians, and pediatric subspecialists should work together to implement standards for health care of children in foster care developed by District II of AAP.
2. All children entering foster care should have an initial physical examination before or soon after placement. This examination should focus on identifying acute and chronic conditions requiring expedient treatment.
3. All children in foster care should receive comprehensive physical and mental health and developmental evaluations within one month of placement.

4. Individual court-approved social service case plans should include the results of physical, mental health, and developmental assessments, and should incorporate the recommendations of health professionals.
5. Pediatricians and child welfare agencies should work together to ensure that children in foster care receive the full range of preventive and therapeutic services needed, and should participate in all federal and state entitlement programs for which they are eligible.
6. Although in placement, the child in foster care requires physical, developmental, and mental health status monitoring more frequently than children living in stable homes with competent parents.
7. Child welfare agencies and health care providers should develop and implement systems to ensure the efficient transfer of physical and mental health information among professionals who treat children in foster care. (AAP, 2002, p. 539)

Although the guidelines do not address all of the issues associated with the health and mental health needs of children entering out-of-home placement, they provide health care practitioners with a place to start in dialoguing with child welfare professionals. Missing from these recommendations is how multiple systems to which the child may be connected (e.g., schools, juvenile justice) interrelate in meeting the health and mental health needs of children in state care.

Case Study

Margaret Cheng, MSW, is a family health practitioner assigned to Johnson family health clinic, located in a poor section of a large metropolitan area in California. The center is a primary care provider for health and mental health screenings of children entering protective services.

Cheng is assigned to a case of neglect involving a ten-year-old Colombian male named Ricky Guadalupe. Until yesterday, Ricky was living with his mother in an apartment in a poor section of town. Child protective services was called after Ricky was picked up by the police and taken to juvenile detention for his participation in a burglary a block away from his home. The police report indicates that this was Ricky's first offense. Notes made by the responding officer state that Ricky had been befriended by older adolescents who said they would pay him if he would allow them to hoist him through a second-story window and, upon entering, unlock the front door to allow the older adolescents to enter the house. Because Ricky was hungry and needed income, he agreed. Police found him eating in the dining room of the burgled house.

A bilingual child protective services social worker interviewed Ricky at the juvenile detention facility. He reported that his father had died six months earlier, and that the last time he saw his mother (three days before) she was very ill. He also indicated that he had not been in school regularly since his father's death, in part because he was waiting to return with his mother to Colombia.

The child protective social worker decided to make a visit with police to Ricky's home. Upon arriving, the worker and police officer noted a stench originating from the apartment. Police officers knocked on the door and, finding no answer, located the apartment manager and asked for entry. They found the apartment littered with animal feces, dirty laundry, rotten half-eaten food, several emaciated cats, and Ricky's mother in a physically deteriorated state in the bedroom. She was rushed by ambulance to the nearest hospital and placed in the intensive care unit.

The juvenile facility transferred physical custody to child protective services for Ricky to be placed in a foster home until his court hearing. The child protective worker, per procedure, brought Ricky to the clinic for a health and mental health screening and assessment. Initial screening indicated that he was malnourished and underweight, showed signs of cognitive delays, had mild asthma, had heart arrhythmia, and was infested with lice.

Appropriate Family Health Practitioner Considerations

The case of Ricky Guadalupe brings up several treatment and systems issues that affect his overall treatment plan. Some of the questions related to treatment include the following: Who has the legal right to make treatment decisions for the child? What is the best course of treatment for the child's malnourishment? What is the best course of treatment for the child's arrhythmia? Does the child's asthma require medication and has he previously received medication for this condition? Are the child's cognitive delays due to a language barrier, disability, social deprivation, or cultural differences? Who (individual and/or system) can authorize treatment? Who (individual and/or system) will pay for treatment? How will treatment information be tracked and monitored? Who (individual and/or system) will authorize follow-up medical care? Questions related to system issues include the following: What is the child's legal status? What multiple service-delivery systems is the child connected to? What are the eligibility restrictions in each of the systems? Are there cooperative agreements between the systems? Do representatives of each interfacing system have to be contacted in order for a complete treatment plan to be developed and implemented?

The child's position relative to the child welfare, juvenile, immigration, and health care delivery systems will directly affect the degree to which Margaret Cheng can do short-term and long-term treatment planning for her client. Also, Cheng's role as the health advocate for the child is directly affected by her professional connections into the overlapping systems of care (juvenile justice, child welfare, immigration, etc.). For her to be successful, she must do coordinated treatment planning, have knowledge of how health-related issues are handled in other care systems, and knowledge of what contributes to the successes and failures when multiple systems are involved. This requires her to have knowledge in her area of expertise as well as in the larger system's dynamics and nuances. Skill development in larger systems requires her to develop a network with staff in interfacing systems, know how to access service delivery in those systems, and anticipate potential complicating factors within those systems. The degree to which she is able to maneuver both within and outside of her own care system will ultimately determine her ability to successfully help clients who are connected to multiple systems.

CONCLUSION

When health practitioners' have to deal with competing systems of care, knowledge related to the structural, functional, and treatment issues associated with each system is vital. Likewise, the primary issue that is faced by family health practitioners has nothing to do with a lack of tested models or professional recommendations regarding how to best work with children in low income families or in out-of-home placement. Rather, it has to do with the moral fortitude of policymakers (governmental and health) to implement recommendations that are already in existence. Reports by the CWLA and the AAP are good starting points in this dialogue since they outline the best practice components in multisystem care.

Delivery of and access to health care for low-income populations has always been politically and socially controversial. In the 1930s, Franklin Roosevelt did not connect health care to social welfare in New Deal programs for much the same reasons Bill Clinton was unable to enact health care reform in the mid-1990s. The similarities included (1) interest groups (medical, business) were against health care reform; (2) Congress was reluctant to take the political risks necessary to seriously consider health care financing and structural realignment (e.g., "socialized medicine" in the 1930s and "universal health care" in the 1990s); and (3) the public was ambivalent about costs associated with reform (access, fee structure, quality of care). Understanding these time-tested roadblocks helps family health practitioners recognize some of the pitfalls in bringing forward health care agendas.

REFERENCES

American Academy of Pediatrics (AAP). (1997). Health care for children in foster care. In *Managed care and children with special health care needs* (pp. 54-58). Elk Grove Village, IL: Author.

American Academy of Pediatrics, Committee on Early Childhood Adoption and Dependent Care (2002). Health care of young children in foster care. *Pediatrics, 109*(3), 536-542.

Bould, S. (1993). Familial caretaking: A middle range definition of family in the context of social policy. *Journal of Family Issues, 14*(1), 133-152.

Charlow, A. (2001). A Minnesota comparative family law symposium: Race, poverty, and neglect. *William Mitchell Law Review, 28*(763), 763-790.

Child Welfare League of America (CWLA). (1988). *Standards for health care for children in out-of-home care.* Washington, DC: Author.

Cohen, N.A. (Ed.). (2000). *Child welfare: A multicultural focus,* Second edition. Needham Heights, MA: Allyn & Bacon.

Crawford, J.M. (1999). Co-parent same-sex couples: From loophole to law. *Families in Society: The Journal of Contemporary Human Services, 80*(3), 271-279.

Crosson-Tower, C. (2001). *Exploring child welfare,* Second edition. Needham Heights, MA: Allyn & Bacon.

Downey, M. (2000/2001). Losing more than time: Incarcerated mothers and the Adoption and Safe Families Act of 1997. *Buffalo Women's Law Journal, 9*(41), 41-49.

English, A., Morreale, M., and Stinnett, A. (1999). *Adolescents in public health insurance programs: Medicaid and CHIP.* Chapel Hill, NC: Center for Adolescent Health and Law.

Geen, R. and Waters, S. (1997). *The impact of welfare reform on child welfare financing.* Series A, No. 4-16, Washington, DC: The Urban Institute.

Greenberg, M. (2001). Welfare reform and devolution. *Brookings Review, 19*(3), 20-26.

Hagen, J. L. (1999). Public welfare and human services: New directions under TANF? *Families in Society: The Journal of Contemporary Human Services, 80*(1), 78-94.

Halfon, N. and Berkowitz, G. (1993). Health care entitlements for children: Providing health services as if children really mattered. In S.G. Goffin and M.A. Jensone (Eds.), *Visions of entitlement: The care and education of America's children* (pp. 175-212). Albany, NY: SUNY Press.

Halfon, N., Inkelas, M., DuPlessis, H., and Newacheck, P.W. (1999). Challenges in securing access to care for children. *Health Affairs, 18*(2), 48-63.

Heck, K.E. and Parker, J.D. (2002). Family strucure, socioeconomic status, and access to health care for children. *Health Services Research, 37*(1), 173-186.

Hutchison, E.D. and Charlesworth, L.W. (2000). Securing the welfare of children: Policies past, present, and future. *Families in Society: The Journal of Contemporary Human Services, 81*(6), 576-597.

Junek, W. and Thompson, A.H. (1999). Self-regulating service delivery systems: A model for children and youth at risk. *The Journal of Behavioral Health Services and Research, 26*(1), 64-79.

Kadushin A. and Martin, J.A. (1988). *Child welfare services,* Fourth edition. Needham Heights, MA: Macmillan Publishing.

Kaiser Family Foundation. (1996). *Medicaid facts: Medicaid and managed care.* Washington, DC: The Kaiser Commission on the Future of Medicaid.

Kronebusch, K. (2001). Children's Medicaid enrollment: The impacts of mandates, welfare reform, and policy. *Journal of Health Politics, Policy, and Law, 26*(6), 1223-1260.

Lewandowski, C.A. and GlenMaye, L.F. (2002). Teams in child welfare settings: Interprofessional collaborative processes. *Families in Society: The Journal of Contemporary Human Services, 83*(3), 245-257.

Machtinger, B. (1999). The U.S. Bureau and Mothers' Pensions Administration, 1912-1930. *Social Service Review, 73*(1), 105-116.

Mason, M.A. and Mauldon, J. (1996). The new stepfamily requires new public policy. *Journal of Social Issues, 52*(3), 11-28.

McLoyd, V. (1998). Socioeconomic disadvantage and child development. *American Psychologist, 53*(2), 185-204.

MorBarak, M.E., Nissly, J.A., and Levin, A. (2001). Antecedents to retention and turnover among child welfare, social work, and other human service employees: What can we learn from past research? A review and metanalysis. *Social Service Review, 75*(4), 625-663.

Morrison, J., Frank, S., Holland, C., and Kates, W. (1999). Emotional development and disorders in young children in the child welfare system. In J. Silver, B. Amster, and T. Haecker (Eds.), *Young children and foster care: A guide for professionals* (pp. 34-64). Baltimore, MD: Paul H. Brookes.

Rosenbach, M. (2001). *Children in foster care: Challenges in meeting their health care needs through Medicaid.* Available online at <www.mathematica-mpr.com/PDFs/fostercarebrief.pdf>.

Rosenbaum, S., Smith, B., Sonosky, C., Repasch, L., and Markus, A. (2001). Children's Health Symposium: Devolution of authority and public health insurance design: National SCHIP study reveals an impact on low-income children. *Houston Journal of Health Law and Policy, 33*(1), 33-61.

Selden, T.M., Banthin, J.S., and Cohen, J.W. (1999). Waiting in the wings: Eligibility and enrollment in the state children's health insurance program. *Health Affairs, 18*(2), 126-133.

Silver, J. (1999). Starting young: Improving children's outcomes. In J. Silver, B. Amster, and T. Haecker (Eds.), *Young children and foster care: A guide for professionals* (pp. 3-32). Baltimore, MD: Paul H. Brookes.

Silver, J., Haecker, T. and Forkey, H. (1999). Health care for young children in foster care. In J. Silver, B. Amster, and T. Haecker (Eds.), *Young children and foster care: A guide for professionals* (pp. 161-195). Baltimore, MD: Paul H. Brookes.

Simms, M.D., Freundlich, M., Battistelli, E.S., and Kaufman, N.D. (1999). Delivering health and mental healthcare services to children in family foster care after welfare and health care reform. *Child Welfare, 78*(1), 166-183.

Simms, M.D. and Halfon, N. (1994). The health care needs of children in foster care: A research agenda. *Child Welfare, 73*(5), 505-524.

Sobel, A. (2000). An exploratory study of resilience using phenomenological methodology: An investigation of protective factors present for Urban Head Start children. Unpublished doctoral dissertation, The George Washington University, Washington, DC.

Sobel, A. and Healy, C. (2001). Fostering health in the foster care maze. *Pediatric Nursing, 27*(5), 493-505.

Stein, T.J. (2000). The Adoption and Safe Families Act: Creating a false dichotomy between parents' and childrens' rights. *Families in Society: The Journal of Contemporary Human Services, 81*(6), 586-600.

Szilagyi, M. (1998). The pediatrician and the child in foster care. *Pediatrics in Review, 19*(20), 39-50.

Takayama, J.I., Wolfe, E. and Coulter, K.P. (1998). Relationships between reason for placement and medical findings among children in foster care. *Pediatrics, 101*(2), 201-208.

Tatara, T. (1993). *Voluntary cooperative information systems (VCIS), characteristic of children in substitute and adoptive care.* Washington, DC: American Public Welfare Association.

Ullman, F. and Hill, I. (2001). Eligibility under state children's health insurance programs. *American Journal of Public Health, 91*(9), 1449-1451.

United States General Accounting Office. (1995). *Health needs of many young children are unknown and unmet* (GAO/HEHS-95-114). Washington, DC: U.S. General Accounting Office.

Waxman, J. and Alker, J. (1996). *The impact of federal welfare reform on Medicaid.* Available online at <www.handsnet.org/medicaid/impact.htm>.

Wolfe, E. and Coulter, K.P. (1998). Relationship between reason for placement and medical findings among children in foster care. *Pediatrics, 101*(2), 201-208.

Wulczyn, F. and Orlebeke, B. (2000). Fiscal reform and managed care in child welfare services. *Policy and Practice of Public Human Services, 58*(3), 26-35.

Wurtele, S.K. (1999). Preventing child maltreatment: Multiple windows of opportunity in the health care system, *Children's Health Care, 28*(2), 151-166.

Yudkowsky, B.K., Cartland, J.D., and Flint, S.S. (1990). Pediatrician participation in Medicaid: 1978-1989. *Pediatrics, 85*, 567-577.

Chapter 11

Homeless Women with Children: Their Health and Implications for Family Health Practice

Susan Talamantes Eggman

I said to my children, "I'm going to work and do everything that I can do to see that you get a good education. I don't ever want you to forget that there are millions of God's children who will not and cannot get a good education, and I don't want you feeling that you are better than they are. For you will never be what you ought to be until they are what they ought to be."

Martin Luther King Jr.
January 7, 1968

INTRODUCTION

People without a place to live or their own address are people and families defined as the homeless. In the United States, every year 2 to 3 million people are homeless (Thompson 2003). Although estimates differ, homeless families make up between 34 and 45 percent of the homeless population (National Center on Family Homelessness 2003; Page, Ainsworth, and Pett 1993). Within the burgeoning population, families with young children are the fastest growing group in the homeless population (The Better Homes Fund 1999; U.S. Department of Health and Human Services 2003; Murrell et al. 2000; Kelly 2001). Homeless families face countless challenges in daily life, including housing, nutrition, and education, but one of most difficult issues for families with children is health and access to health care.

This chapter is about health and implications for health care in home-less families.

Case Study: Erica and Her Family

Let's use an example to make the model and population come to life. This is a fictitious case based on the literature and demographics of homeless families. For the purpose of exploration, let's say a social worker at a center for homeless and poor families that provides free, but limited, medical and dental clinic treatment receives a referral to see Erica, a twenty-eight-year-old single mother. She has a six-month-old baby named Justice who suffers from chronic ear infections that make him cry constantly. She also has a four-year-old girl named Karma and a seven-year-old boy named John. Karma and Justice share the same father but John has a different father. Erica has never been married. Erica and her children currently reside in a shelter for women and children.

More information about demographics, etiology, and policy issues are necessary prior to undertaking any assessment and intervention. This chapter will include a look at homeless families, reasons for homelessness, health care policy, and health care issues related to homelessness and Erica's case study. All of this is in context of think-ing about using the family health approach as a means practice in working with homeless families.

HOMELESS FAMILIES: A DEFINITION

The homeless, by definition, are a group of people difficult to track. The usual means of "counting" people defy researchers and surveyors when it comes to the homeless. Homeless people do not have homes to which surveys can be sent, phones to call, or the e-mail addresses necessary to be on mailing lists. Homeless families are on the move or staying in a variety of places. Not all families utilize or have access to the shelter system in which counting is most often done. The urban homeless are more likely to live in shelters, whereas rural homeless are more likely to live in tents, garages, or doubled up in some other way with family and friends. Previously, the "homeless issue" existed primarily in major cities. This is no longer the case. A national survey conducted by the Urban Institute, found 71 percent of homeless clients live in major cities, 20 percent live in the suburbs, and 9 percent live in rural areas (Burt et al. 1999). Keep in mind the problems inherent in counting people without homes or addresses.

Years of working with this new population have painted a picture of the "average" homeless family. The average homeless family consists of a single mother with two young children under the age of six (The Better Homes Fund 1999; Page, Ainsworth, and Pett 1993). One large-scale research project of shelters found that 94 percent of children entering shelters were under the age of five and in the care of their mothers (Lewis and Meyers 1989). In addition, homeless women are more likely to be pregnant or to have had a child in the past year than women who are not homeless. She generally has less than a high school education and minimal or no job skills (da Costa Nunez 1996; Murrell et al. 2000). The homeless family's average annual income is less than $8,000 (The Better Homes Fund 1999).

Research suggests that as children, 63 percent of homeless women experienced physical abuse, and 42 percent experienced sexual abuse (National Center on Family Homelessness 2003). That less than half of homeless mothers have completed high school is not unforeseen given their backgrounds. When combining childhood abuse with their experience as adults, 92 percent of homeless mothers have experienced physical or sexual assault (The Better Homes Fund 1999).

Domestic violence is a problem frequently associated with homeless women. Domestic violence is another source of stress and trauma in the lives of homeless women that reduces their ability to be effective parents and can result in behavioral and emotional problems for their children (National Center on Family Homelessness 2003; Passero Rabideau and Toro 1997). It is humbling to think that mothers are often faced with the choice between continued abuse for themselves or their children or resorting to the uncertain and dangerous life in the shelter system or on the streets.

Many women who are homeless were in the foster care system as children and youth (da Costa Nunez 1996). One study found that one-third of homeless women in their sample had been raised outside of their parents' care, and 61 percent of their own children were either in foster care or had been in foster care in the past (Zlotnick, Robertson, and Wright 1999). Placement in foster care is one of only two childhood risk factors that predict family homelessness as an adult (The Better Homes Fund 1999). Parenting development might be in order in any kind of intervention since these women might have limited examples of positive parenting.

WHY ARE FAMILIES HOMELESS?

Beginning in the 1980s, homelessness became a risk factor for families living in poverty (Duchon 1998). The policies of the 1980s were disastrous to poor and working families. Since 1980 there has been a 500 percent increase in family homelessness (Nunez 2001). Trade and production jobs that once supported a family no longer exist. Jobs that are available for those without degrees or experience are largely within the low-paying service industry. Combined with the dwindling job market, the past two decades have seen income or assistance in the form of public benefits decrease significantly. This will continue even more noticeably as programs are shifted from the federal to state level. In addition, those with limited income find it harder to locate affordable housing. In some cities there is a 0 percent occupancy rating! Within the past two decades there has been a significant decrease in the number of affordable housing units. Families with children have some of the most pressing housing needs. Children who live in substandard housing or no housing at all experience conditions that put them at risk for health problems and injury.

Between 1973 and 1993, more than 2 million low-rent housing units disappeared from the market. At the same time, the number of low-income renters increased by nearly 5 million (U.S. Department of Health and Human Services 2003). Logically thinking, lack of affordable housing is a leading cause of homelessness. In 2000, housing requests went up in 76 percent of the cities surveyed (U.S. Conference of Mayors 2000). A recent report found that a family of four, making $38,000 a year, which is double the poverty rate, does not have enough to provide the basic necessities of housing, food, and health care (National Center for Children in Poverty 2002).

One ethnographic study of homeless women revealed that external factors such as the reduction in aid and the larger effects of the economy most often lead to women being unable to pay rent. Reduction in aid and the increase in the cost of living forced women to pay the same amount of rent with a more limited budget (Thrasher and Mowbray 1995). A study of pregnant women and parenting homeless women in San Francisco cited the following reasons for their homelessness: lack of finances, domestic violence, loss of a job or a partner's job, housing eviction, and substance abuse issues (Murrell et al. 2000)

The most common reasons cited for homelessness fall into two groups: internal and external. *Internal* refers to an issue with the individual, and *external* refers to a problem outside of the individual. It is limiting to think of these as "either/or" categories. For example, a housing eviction, generally thought of as a problem with a person, could easily come about because of issues such as gentrification. As the housing market continues to go up, landlords can without a doubt charge more money for the same apartment that has suddenly become prime real estate. Similarly, houses that have once been rentals can attain high prices in a limited sellers' market. So although we might normally attribute an eviction to an internal variable such as drug abuse or poor money management, it is increasingly important to look at the issue holistically and in context. Similarly, an issue of substance abuse initially looks to be an internal issue of homelessness and might well be. However, lack of available substance abuse treatment, especially for women with children, might also be considered an external issue. Although an internal factor such as mental illness might lead to homelessness, it can also be argued that living in the stressful conditions of homelessness can also produce emotional disorder (Passero Rabideau and Toro 1997).

POVERTY AND HOMELESSNESS

Although many issues are associated with homeless families, the undeniable constant factor is poverty. Homelessness is a process of poverty (Lewis and Meyers 1989). Poverty can be visualized as the bookends to the story of homeless families; homelessness is only one part of the sequence of being poor. Many homeless families have experienced generational poverty and most have been poor prior to their current episode of homelessness. Families remain homeless for an average of five months per episode of homelessness (U.S. Conference of Mayors 2000). After homelessness families seldom transition to a life of luxury, but instead return to previous levels of poverty and minimal living. Moreover, families who have been homeless previously are at the highest risk for being homeless again, and 34 percent of families who are currently homeless have been homeless before (Burt et al. 1999).

Children in the United States are almost twice as likely as any other age group to live in poverty (Lu 2002). Recent data clearly reveal that the first years of life are more important for a child's emotional and intellectual development than had previously been thought. This new information significantly increases the urgency of addressing one of the most important risk factors that can impede young children's development: poverty. In the United States, 5 million children live in extreme poverty, with their parents earning $8,000 a year or less, a 17 percent increase since 2000 (Lu 2002). The 2.1 million poor children under the age of three face a greater likelihood of impaired development than children with adequate resources. Increased exposure to a number of factors associated with poverty include inadequate nutrition, environmental toxins, diminished interaction due to maternal depression, trauma and abuse, lower quality child care, and parental substance abuse. All of these risk factors are associated with impaired brain development (Song and Lu 2002). Impaired development as a child reduces the chance for a healthy, prosperous future as an adult.

Because of the history of poverty, abuse, and instability, homeless families often find themselves without much external support. One task force found that almost half the woman interviewed could not name a support person and many named their minor child as their sole support (Regional Task Force on the Homeless 2003). Contrary to the claim of no support, other research indicates that family and friends are often available emotionally but are unable to help financially or with shelter as they themselves are living in tenuous or restrictive living situations (Nunez 2001). What can break the cycle? Women identify child care, transportation, job training, placement help, and obtaining their GED as services or supports essential in achieving long-term employment (National Center on Family Homelessness 2003).

Remember the image of poverty as bookends around the story of homeless families. Many things such as injury or sickness can easily push a poor family over the edge into homelessness. Some estimate that for every homeless family there are two or three families who are on the verge of homelessness due to unstable living conditions (Regional Task Force on the Homeless 2003). These families often need similar supports to maintain housing and stability, which those who are currently homeless need. Without lasting and effective intervention, homelessness is a recurring theme for many of the poorest families.

HEALTH CARE POLICY TO HOMELESS FAMILIES

Prior to the 1980s, the homeless were thought to be a fairly heterogonous group of people: mostly men whose life conditions or lifestyle had led to their descent to the streets. During the 1980s, opinion on this began to change as the homeless population began to grow and diversify. Although it was easier to think of healthy men on the street, it was more difficult to see women, children, and families on the streets and in shelters. Organizations responded and began providing food, clothing, and shelter. One issue that was not being addressed was one of health care needs. When it was established that the homeless are at greater risks of health issues, knowing minor health care issues can develop into major issues, it was determined something had to be done (Stephens 1991).

The Stewart B. McKinney Homeless Assistance Act was signed into law in 1987. This act supplied federal funding for homeless health care to communities in a comprehensive manner. It was assumed that because the homeless population was no longer the homogenized population it was once envisioned to be their health care needs would be equally as diverse (Stephens 1991). There was also acknowledgement given that how and where the health care was delivered was as important as what was given. Here is a policy statement excerpt from the Government office of Health Care for the Homeless:

> There is a critical need for programs that are specifically targeted to provide health care to this underserved segment of society. Although homeless programs have much in common with other community-based providers of care to underserved populations, it is also markedly different. Homeless individuals suffer from health care problems at more than double the rate of individuals with stable housing. This phenomenon is exacerbated by the multiple barriers that homeless people experience in trying to access health care. Homeless people frequently find that a lack of transportation and the limited hours of service

present barriers to accessing mainstream service. When home-less individuals do attempt to access services, they routinely do not have the necessary financial resources (health insurance, Medicaid, etc.) to pay for the care. Additionally, many homeless individuals have significant mental health and/or substance abuse problems. As a result, they become increasingly disenfran-chised from mainstream services and are frequently distrustful of traditional health care and social service systems. (U.S. De-partment of Health and Human Services 2003)

As a result, the model for health care delivery that has been developed is one of community collaboration and outreach. As more care was delivered, it was discovered that more and more children were being served by these funded community agencies. In 1992 a federal pro-gram named the Outreach and Primary Health Services for Homeless Children Program (HCHC) was added as an addendum.

The homeless children program is a grant program that recognizes the importance of collaboration between community agencies. The program funds innovative and creative programs for outreach, refer-ral, and health services for homeless children and children at risk of homelessness. There is a strong focus on preventative care and com-prehensive primary care services (U.S. Department of Health and Human Services 2001). Grants are provided to agencies, and not all services will be provided by one grantee but from a number of collab-orative programs (U.S. Department of Health and Human Services 2003). This idea for a multidisciplinary collaborative approach stems from a four-year pilot study conducted by the Robert Woods Johnson Foundation and the Pew Charitable Trusts foundation. The study con-firmed that homeless individuals and families have more compro-mised health than the general population and without specific inter-vention will fall through the cracks more often than not. Heartening findings suggest that people can be reached and treated by this multidisciplinary outreach type program (U.S. Department of Health and Human Services 2001).

Although the outreach collaborative model is an innovative step, multiple barriers to health care still exist, stemming from the condi-tion of homelessness itself. Homeless people often have a lack of in-formation about the programs, have difficulty completing applica-tions and proving eligibility, lack transportation, and, of course, have many other priorities. In addition, not having a place to live makes compliance virtually impossible for things such as medications every four hours, bed rest, elevating a limb, and obtaining and refrigerating medications, among other factors (Clement 2003; Gale 2003). Compounding the difficulties with homelessness and health care, there are always various system barriers that impact the delivery of services. Although the idea of outreach, and collaboration are crucial, it can also lead to fragmentation of services and lack of accountability and resources (Gale 2003)

HEALTH AND HEALTH CARE ISSUES
FOR HOMELESS FAMILIES

America spends more on health care per capita, yet millions are without health care insurance and denied the most basic of health care services (Wood 1992). Although poor families have many of the same health issues and complications as homeless families, quantitative measures show homeless families scoring worse (Duchon 1998). Health care, when obtained, is often too little too late. Routine preventative care such as annual checkups and immunizations are not a high priority for a family that has to find safe shelter for a night and food for a day (Duchon 1998).

Simply put, homelessness makes children sick. Without access to health care, chronic illness goes without detection and treatment until they become emergencies (Homelessness and Family Trauma 2003). Researchers have identified homelessness as a predictor for specific childhood illnesses. Clement (2003) identified the following as health issues for which homeless children are specifically at risk: poor nutrition, poor dental care, anemia, infections, asthma, lack of immunizations, growth and development problems, mental health conditions, and other issues related to lack of a safe stable environment, for example, accidents, skin conditions, lead poisonings, and multiple types of abuse (Clement 2003). Homeless children are in fair to poor health twice as often as other children whose families earn more than $35,000 annually. They have higher rates of low birth rate, and special care needs after birth four times more often than other children. Homeless children also have higher rates of acute illnesses, twice as many ear infections, five times the diarrhea and stomach problems, are four times as likely to be asthmatic, and go hungry at twice the rate of other children (The Better Homes Fund 1999). Looking at this picture, it would be hard to dispute to detrimental impact of homelessness on children's health.

Although health is an issue for all children living in poverty, homeless children fare worse than their low-income housed counterparts (Duchon 1998). A study of a school-based comprehensive health care program found that homeless children were 2.5 times as likely to have health problems and three times as likely to have severe health problems as housed poor children (Berti, Zylbert, and Rolnitzky 2001). Homeless children are twice as likely to experience hunger and four times as likely to have delayed development than children with stable housing (National Coalition for the Homeless 2001). Homeless babies show slower development than other children as well as mental and emotional health issues that require professional mental health care (The Better Homes Fund 1999). As stated previously, homeless women are more likely to be pregnant or have had a baby in the past year than other woman. Babies are born at higher risk with general health conditions, low birth weight, and with mother's who have had minimal prenatal care. In addition, these often fragile infants leave the hospital and go to a shelter.

Another population of children that bears mentioning here is homeless youth. These are young people who have been abandoned or discarded; have left the foster care system; or for other reasons find themselves on the streets. They have high rates of victimization, both before and after becoming homeless. They also have high rates of HIV and AIDS, STDs, and other health care issues that have become chronic due to lack of preventive health care. As a group they suffer from high rates of substance abuse and mental health issues. Many of these youth have suffered severe abuses in their family of origin, and they are at high rates of revicitimization on the streets (Ryan et al. 2000). Developmentally, adolescent youth are experiencing sexual maturity and are at high risk for pregnancy. Many of these young people will find themselves pregnant and become young homeless families.

Although perhaps not always the case, it is safe to propose that hunger is a common occurrence of homelessness. Hunger and poor nutrition are common experiences for homeless children, and inadequate diets contribute to unhealthy growth and development. Due to the transient nature of homeless families, children tend to fall behind in school and often experience developmental delays. Nutrition is one of the important, and certainly addressable, variables in healthy brain development in children (Song and Lu 2002). In the Mayors survey, 86 percent of the cities surveyed reported increases in families' request for emergency food (U.S. Conference of Mayors 2000).

One study examining the associations between food insufficiency, family income, and health for preschool and school-aged children found that poor children are more often hungry children. In addition, this study concluded that children with food insuffiency have a low health status and are more likely to experience such complications as frequent colds, and more stomach and headaches than children with enough to eat (Alaimo et al. 2001). For both preschool and school-aged children, hunger is found to be a predictor of chronic illness and behavior problems (Weinrab et al. 2002).

Dental health is a major problem for homeless children. There are fewer resources for dental care than for medical care for low-income and homeless populations. One study found that 95 percent of pre-school-age children had not seen a dentist (Clement 2003). Although seeing a dentist is important, many homeless children find it impossible to maintain such good dental hygiene as brushing and flossing. This neglect can lead to cavities, infections, and abscesses, which can be compounded by a poor diet. A painful mouth can make eating problematic, especially healthy food such as fruits and vegetables, which can further compromise nutrition. Moreover, a mouth full of crooked, discolored, missing, or infected teeth makes a homeless child an even greater target for ridicule and isolation from peers (Children's Defense Fund 2003).

Homeless mothers have higher rates of depression and anxiety than do their nonhomeless counterparts (San Agustin et al. 1999). Maternal depression is linked to lack of brain development in children under three (Song and Lu 2002). Despite any good intentions, a mother who is depressed has less internal resources to comfort and nurture her children. This inability to nurture cannot help but negatively impact a child's development. One of the most important risk factors for children is parent psychopathology. One of the strongest predictors for a child's healthy attachment and emotional development is their mother's level of distress (Homelessness and Family Trauma 2003). The accumulation of multiple sources of stress can lead to decreased coping, and increase the likelihood of psychological distress for these young mothers (Passero Rabideau and Toro 1997).

Homeless children are under an inordinate amount of stress and worry. They worry about themselves as well as their families. It is routine for homeless children to have mothers who have experienced domestic violence as well as mental illness and addictions. Subsequently, children live in a continuous state of stress that can have effects on their emotional and cognitive development (Homelessness and Family Trauma 2003). Homeless children experience more mental health problems such as anxiety, depression, and withdrawal than housed children (National Coalition for the Homeless 2001).

Poor living conditions make children and families especially vulnerable to accidents and injury (Clement 2003). Children living in shelters, doubled or tripled up with friends and family, or living in parks, cars, or other public places cannot help but be exposed to more danger than children living in a stable situation. Burns, broken bones, bumps and bruises, although common for all children, can be part of daily life for a homeless child. And, finally, asthma is at an almost epidemic rate for homeless children. More than 4.4 million children in the United States are affected by asthma. This rate is double what it was ten years ago. In addition to the genetic and allergy factors associated with asthma, it can also be triggered by environmental factors such as air pollution, animal hair, dust mites, and cigarette smoke (Children's Defense Fund 2003).

After examining all of the health care issues faced specifically by homeless children and families, keep in mind that 58 percent of homeless children are without health care insurance (Berti, Zylbert, and Rolnitzky 2001). So while having higher health care needs, they have fewer resources than other children. Given this picture, it is crucial to have a theoretical roadmap for guidance when working with health care for a homeless family.

Family Health Approach

The emerging family health approach of practice is a good fit in working with and understanding homeless families. It is limiting to think of working with homeless families and their health care needs from an exclusively physical standpoint. To work with illness in isolation from social, psychological, and environmental factors is generally restrictive, but with homeless families, it is increasingly so. The family health model focuses on "a holistic well-being of the family and its members" (Yuen 1999, p. 17). Inherent in homeless families is that the entire well-being of the family is at high risk. It would be seemingly impossible to look only at the family system and not take into account that family health approaches focus on human behavior and the social environment (Yuen 2003). And, finally, to not think about macro complications and implications in assessing and intervening with families would be extraordinarily limited. Social workers need to think not only about helping people who have slipped through the increasingly large cracks, but also about how to join with others to seal the cracks to prevent others from slipping.

Definition of the Family

The family health model definition of family is inclusive of many types of family. Although the family of origin is the most common in thinking of families, it is limiting when thinking of the realities of those who find themselves of the streets. A family is a system of two or more persons, tied together by blood, marriage, adoption, or by those who commit to each other for the basic and common purpose of "promoting the economic, physical, mental, emotional, social, cultural, and spiritual growth and development of the unit and each of its members" (Yuen, Skibinski, and Pardeck 2003, p. 203).

Although this chapter discusses more traditional conceptualizations, when working with the homeless population, social workers will find the family health approach useful in assessing family systems. A family might be a group of adolescents that live and function together and define themselves as a family. The family health approach is conceptualized across the dimensions of nature, structure, and function (Yuen, Skibinski, and Pardeck 2003; Yuen 1999).

- *Nature:* The family is the primary unit upon which society is based. The nature of a family is its ability to build upon the characteristics and abilities of the individual members for the good of the whole. A question to ask is, What is the nature of this family?
- *Structure:* Whereas nature speaks to a family's personality, the structure of a family speaks to how it does those things. The

structure of a family is the sum of its interactions with each other and the environment. In systems theory, repeated transactions form patterns. And repeated patterns become the foundation for a family's function.

- *Function:* Family function comprises the activities necessary for realizing the family's common purpose to promote economic, physical, mental, emotional, social, cultural, and spiritual growth of each of its members and its self.
- *Family life cycle:* The family health approach incorporates the understanding of families in different stages of the life cycle. A family with young children might have very different needs than a family comprised of adolescent children. This is certainly relevant when thinking about families negotiating such resources as school, health care, transportation, and general safety needs of family members at varying stages of development and composition.
- *Social construction:* The family health model also looks at the social construction of family. This suggests that we must depend on the family to provide their definition of what family means to them. Although society and even the U.S. Supreme Court might provide legal guidelines in thinking about concepts such as nature, structure, and function, the family in question is really the expert on their members and their goals and dreams for their family's holistic well-being and fit with their environment.
- *Ecological and systems perspective:* This is perhaps the most pertinent concept of the family health approach when engaging with homeless families. Ecological systems perspective at its core is concerned with, "the growth, development, and potentialities of human beings and with the properties of their environments that support or fail to support the expressions of human potential" (Germain 1979, p. 7). At its essence, the ecological systems perspective is concerned with the adaptation of both people and their environments. The combined perspective focuses on the transactions and adaptations of people in their environments, and makes this a perspective that can intervene from the micro- to macrolevel. Using this perspective, social workers assess the habitat and niche of individuals and families in their human quest for community. *Habitat* can be thought of as housing or the environment in which people live, and *niche* refers to a

unique place, position, competence, function, or ability (Robbins, Chatterjee, Canda 1998). Encountering a homeless family is encountering a family in crisis of habitat and niche. If these two concepts are visualized as core to a person's or family's holistic well-being, it is clear that interventions and supports will be necessary across systems. How might one think about assessing and strengthening a family, or their environments, transactions, adaptive ability, and overall well-being, thereby strengthening the overall community or habitat for us all?

- *Biopsychosocial:* The idea of continuum is key and inclusive for the biopsychosocial way of thinking about family health. All of the previously mentioned components of family and environment are now assessed across a family's or individual's biological, psychological, and social functioning.

Case Study: Erica and Her Family

Using the family health approach as a guide, the social worker sets out to do a holistic assessment with Erica. The doctor has determined that Justice needs to have surgery on his ears, as they have been chronically infected. Because of the chronic infections, Justice's eardrums continued to rupture and now require surgery. Erica could never completely cure her baby's ear infections. The medication prescribed needed to be kept in a refrigerator and she was not allowed to use the shelter refrigerator for personal items. Also, transportation to see a doctor and have prescriptions filled has been difficult. The physician would like the social worker to see if Erica and her children are eligible for insurance and to obtain stable housing for the postoperative care Justice will require.

In the assessment the social worker discovered that Erica did not finish high school. Her family was poor and moved frequently. Erica had trouble keeping up with her studies and fitting in at each new school. When she was sixteen she dropped out and got a job at a fast-food restaurant. She met and moved in with John's father when she was eighteen. He had a construction job that paid fairly well. He drank a lot and would use cocaine on the weekends. His drug use eventually became out of control and he lost their apartment. Erica stayed with her sister after that. Her sister helped with child care for John, as she had two children of her own and was on welfare. They made do in the two-bedroom apartment.

Erica could not afford a place of her own even though she worked full-time at the fast-food restaurant. She then met Karma and Justice's father Jordan, who was abusive from the minute she moved in. For a while, Erica went back and forth from Jordan's house to her sister's house, but her sister, married now, was moving in with her husband's family. Erica became pregnant and couldn't afford to move out. Erica and her children left a couple of times and stayed at a domestic violence shelter. Finally, after a bad beating while pregnant, Erica left Jordan for what she hopes is good.

Erica stayed at a women's shelter for a while; after the baby came she went to a family shelter, where she is currently staying. The conditions are very crowded and she and her children have limited privacy. There might be trouble with her staying there now since the baby is crying so much and requiring so much of her attention. She feels overwhelmed and depressed. She hasn't been able to supervise John and he got into some trouble by throwing rocks and fighting with other children. The house manager made a referral to child protective services and Erica is dreading the visit. She has prided herself on never losing her children to the foster care system. She spent some time there as a child when her family was unable to care for her and her sister. Erica was abused in foster care and states she will do anything to prevent having her children "go into one of those heartless houses."

Her oldest son John has attention-deficit disorder. He has been on medication, but Erica has not been able to get the medication regularly since leaving Jordan. John has also struggled with asthma for years. She knows he is behind in school. Karma hasn't been tested, but Erica is concerned she might be a little delayed. Her speech is still minimal and she does not know her colors. A few months ago, a stray dog in a park where they stayed for a few nights bit Karma. She now seems to cry all the time and Erica reports that she is unusually frightened of everything.

When the social worker asks Erica about her own health, she becomes tearful. She states she thinks she is healthy, but feels very tired, overwhelmed, and irritable. She says she feels helpless and as if she and her children are living a nightmare. She acknowledges that she vacillates between yelling at her children and ignoring them. She says she thinks they have all become invisible and she worries they will just "disappear."

When the social worker asks about family, it is discovered whom she views as in and out of her family system and habitat. She does not consider her children's fathers as family as they did not meet her criteria. She is close to her sister, and states they have always been there for each other, "no matter what." Her mother died of an overdose when Erica was in high school. She is fairly close with her father. He is emotionally supportive but is unable to help financially. His chronic breathing problems that impact his ability to work have now rendered him fairly disabled. He does not have a car and lives in a senior living supported-housing building about an hour away. It was the closest place he could find. She talks to him on the phone but does not get to visit often. Family has always been important to her, but they had never had much so she did not have any expectations that they could help her financially. Erica states that she does not really have any other supports. She knows some people in the shelter but nobody she considers her friend. She states she has always been shy and somewhat of a loner, never feeling as if she fit in.

After the social worker has gathered all of the initial information, the worker sets out to make sense of it and apply the created model of intervention. The following are sample questions that can be asked about Erica, her

family, their environment, and the interactions and transactions in and between systems from the family health approach:

- Who is involved, from the immediate to the extended environment?
- Who or what makes up the habitat?
- What kind of niche does Erica and her family occupy?
- How does the family perceive themselves and their niche? How do
  others perceive them?
- Does their niche positively or negatively affect them in relation to other
  people and institutions in the environment?
- What kind of stresses, recent and accumulative, has the family experi-
  enced?
- What kind of coping strategies have they been using and how suc-
  cessful are the strategies in the current situation?
- What are the strengths of Erica and her family?
- What are the stages and or extent of development for Erica and her
  family? Think of development broadly defined here, it may include life
  cycle stages, physiological growth, and psychological and social de-
  velopment.
- What are the nature, structure, function, and construction of family for
  Erica?
- What issues can be identified across the biopsychosocial continuum
  of health? (Adapted from Yuen 2003, pp. 21-22.)

IMPLICATIONS

Although it seems that family homelessness and its multitude of
corresponding issues would be an area of intense interest for health
care providers, policymakers, and social workers, little attention has
been focused on the issue (da Costa Nunez 1996, Thrasher and
Mowbray 1995). The issue of homeless women with children is particularly relevant to the social work profession as social workers have
always been at the forefront of providing services to the most vulnerable populations (Holloway 1991). Although social work has its roots
in working with the poor and disenfranchised, new studies say social
workers have gone away from working with the poor and homeless
population (Perry 2003)

Due to the recent decline of our economy, decreasing jobs, and
more lower paying jobs in the service sector, combined with the onset
of time limits of Temporary Assitance for Needy Families (TANF),
the number of homeless families can be expected to increase. Picking
up any newspaper in the country tells the story of job losses and an

overwhelming housing shortage and health care crisis. The stories do not often tell the tale of those for whom this has the most severe impact. It is imperative that we develop models to maintain family health.

Questions

1. In thinking about providing comprehensive health care to homeless children, what would be the benefits and detriments to having a health care facility at a school?
2. How might one go about surveying homeless families about their health care needs in one's area? What might be some problems to overcome in accessing this population?
3. In thinking about Erica and her family, how do you see external and internal factors impacting her homelessness?
4. What would it take to create communities of opportunity rather than communities of risk for families with the fewest resources? How might using the family health approach enable you to conceptualize communities of opportunities?

REFERENCES

Alaimo, K., Olson, C.M., Frongillo, E.A., and Briefel R.R. (2001). Food insufficiency, family income, and health in United States preschool and school aged children. *American Journal of Public Health* 91(5), 781-786.

Berti, L.C., Zylbert, S., and Rolnitzky, L. (2001). Comparison of health status for children using a school-based health center for comprehensive care. *Journal of Pediatric Health Care* 15(5), 244-250.

The Better Homes Fund (1999). Homeless children: America's new outcasts. Newton, MA: Author.

Burt, M.A., Laudan, A.Y., Douglas, T., Valente, J., Lee, E., and Iwen, B. (1999). *Homelessness: Programs and the people they serve.* Findings of the National Survey of Homeless Assistance Providers and Clients: Urban Institute.

Children's Defense Fund (2003). Every child deserves a healthy start. Oral Health Online. Available online at <www.childrensdefense.org/hs_tp_oralhlth.php>.

Clement, M. (2003). *Children at health risk.* Malden, MA: Blackwell Publishing.

da Costa Nunez, R. (1996). *The new poverty: Homeless families in America.* New York: Insight Books, Plenum Press.

Duchon, L. (1998). *Families and their health care after homelessness: Opportunities for improving access.* New York: Garland Publishing.

Gale, K. (2003). *Holes in the safety net: Mainstream systems and homelessness.* Charles and Helen Schwab Foundation. San Mateo, California.

Germain, C. (1979). *Introduction: Ecology and social work.* In C. Germain (Ed.), *Social Work Practice: People and Environments: An Ecological Perspective* (pp. 1-22). New York: Columbia University Press.

Holloway, S. (1991). Homeless people. In A. Gitterman (Ed.), *Handbook of social work practice with vulnerable populations* (pp. 584-617). New York: Columbia University Press.

Homelessness and Family Trauma: The Case for Early Intervention (2003). Healing Hands: HCH Clinicians Network 7(2), 1-6.

Kelly, E. (2001). Assessment of dietary intake of preschool children living in homeless shelters. *Applied Nursing Research* 14(3), 146-154.

Lewis, M.R. and Meyers, A.F. (1989). The growth and development status of homeless children entering shelters in Boston. *Public Health Reports* 104(3), 247-4.

Lu, H.H. (2002). *Low income children in the United States: A brief demographic profile.* National Center for Children in Poverty. Mailman School of Public Health, Columbia University.

Murrell, N., Scherzer, T., Ryan, M., Frappier, N., Abrams, A., and Roberts, C. (2000). The aftercare project: An intervention for homeless childbearing families. *Family and Community Health* 23(i3), 17-24.

National Center for Children in Poverty (2003). Fact sheet. Mailman School of Public Health, Columbia University. Available online at <www.nccp.org/fact.html>.

National Center on Family Homelessness (2003). Public education and policy. Fact sheet. Available online at <www.familyhomelessness.org/edu_policy.html>.

National Coalition for the Homeless (2001). Homeless families with children. Fact sheet #7. Washington, DC: Author.

Nunez, R. (2001). Family homelessness in New York City: A case study. *Political Science Quarterly* 116(3), 367-379.

Page, A., Ainsworth, A., and Pett, M. (1993). Homeless families and their children's health problems a Utah urban experience. *Western Journal of Medicine* 138(1), 30-36.

Passero Rabideau, J.M. and Toro, P.A. (1997). Social and environmental predictors of adjustment in homeless children. *Journal of Prevention and Intervention in the Community,* 15(2), 1-17.

Perry, R. (2003). Who wants to work with the poor and homeless? *Journal of Social Work Education* 39(2), 321-341.

Regional Task Force on the Homeless, San Diego (2003). Families with children and homelessness. Available online at <www.co.san-diego.ca.us/rtfh/families. html>.

Robbins, S., Chatterjee, P., and Canda, E. (1998). *Contemporary human behavior theory: A critical perspective for social work.* Boston: Allyn & Bacon.

Ryan, D.K., Kilmer, R.P., Cauce, A.M., Watanabe, H., and Hoyt, D.R. (2000). Psychological consequences of child maltreatment in homeless adolescents: Untangling the unique effects of maltreatment an family environment. *Child Abuse and Neglect* 24(3), 333-352.

San Agustin, M., Cohen, P., Rubin, D., Cleary, S.D., Erickson, C.J., and Allen, J.K. (1999). The Montefiore Community Children's project: A controlled study of cognitive and emotional problems of homeless mothers and children. *Journal of Urban Health* 76(1), 39-50.

Song, Y. and Lu, I-I. (2002). Early childhood poverty: A statistical profile. National Center for Children in Poverty. Mailman School of Public Health, Columbia University.

Stephens, D., Dennis, E., Toomer, M., and Holloway (1991). The diversity of case management needs for the care of homeless persons. *Public Health Reports* 106(1), 15-17.

Thompson, T.G. (2003). Ending chronic homelessness: Strategies for action. U.S. Department of Health and Human Services. Available online at <http://aspe.hhs.gov/homeless/index.shtml>.

Thrasher, S. and Mowbray, C. (1995). A strengths perspective: An ethnographic study of homeless women with children. *Health and Social Work* 20(2), 93-99.

U.S. Conference of Mayors (2000). *A status report on hunger and homelessness in America's cities.* Washington, DC: U.S. Conference of Mayors.

U.S. Department of Health and Human Services (2003). Health care for the homeless: The face of homelessness. Available online at <http://bphc.hrsa.gov/hchirc/about/face_homelessness.htm>.

U.S. Department of Health and Human Services, Bureau of Primary Care (2001). Outreach and primary services for homeless children. Available online at <www.bphc.hrsa.gov/programs/HCHCPProgramInfo.HTM>.

Weinrab, L., Wehler, C., Perloff, J., Scott, R., Hosmer, D., Sagor, L., and Gundersen, C. (2002). Hunger: Its impact on children's health and mental health. *Pediatrics,* 110(4), 41.

Wood, D. (1992). *Delivering health care to homeless persons: The diagnosis and management of medical and mental conditions.* New York: Springer Publishing.

Yuen, F.K.O. (1999). The properties of the family health approach. In J.T. Pardeck and F.K.O. Yuen (Eds.), *Family health: A holistic approach to social work practice* (pp. 17-28). Binghamton, NY: The Haworth Press.

Yuen, F.K.O. (2003). Critical concerns for family health practice. In F.K.O. Yuen, G. Skibinski, and J. Pardeck (Eds.), *Family health social work practice: A knowledge and skills casebook* (pp. 19-36). Binghamton, NY: The Haworth Press.

Yuen, F.K.O., Skibinski, G., and Pardeck, J. (2003). *Family health social work practice: A knowledge and skills casebook.* Binghamton, NY: The Haworth Press.

Zlotnick, C., Robertson, M.J., and Wright, M.A. (1999). The impact of foster care and other out-of-home placement on homeless women and their children. *Child Abuse and Neglect* 23(11), 1057-1068.

Chapter 12

The Neighborhood As a Resource for Family Health Social Work Practice

Nicole Nicotera

The neighborhood in which the child lives is an early and major arena for exploration and social interaction, and serves as a setting for the physical and emotional development of the child. (Garbarino et al. 1992, p. 202)

INTRODUCTION

Yuen (2003) states that "family health social work practitioners should develop the ability to understand the dynamics within and among . . . ecosystem networks to form the basis for designing proper interventions" (p. 21). This chapter examines the dynamics of the neighborhood ecosystem as a resource for family health social work practice with children and families. Part one of the chapter discusses the neighborhood as both a habitat and a niche. Part two presents a review of the literature that exposes the importance of neighborhoods for children and families as viewed through an adult's worldview. The literature is summarized in light of questions suggested by Yuen (2003) that are aimed at increasing the family health social work practitioner's ability to understand the dynamics within and among ecosystems. These questions are as follows:

1. "Who is involved in the ecosystem from the immediate to the extended environments? Who makes up the habitat?"
2. "What kinds of niches do individuals or families occupy? How do the individuals or families perceive themselves and their niches in their environments?"

3. "How have these niches positively and negatively affected the individuals or families in relation to other people and institutions in the environment?" (Yuen, 2003, p. 21)

Given the marginalization of children's voices in the research and other literature on neighborhoods, part three reviews research studies in which the child's worldview is paramount. These studies are also summarized in terms of the three questions just stated. Part four presents a case study of a child's neighborhood as niche and habitat for a discussion of assessment and intervention for the family health social work practitioner. Part five provides a concluding discussion, learning exercises, discussion questions, and recommended readings.

PART ONE:
UNDERSTANDING THE NEIGHBORHOOD
AS HABITAT AND NICHE

Neighborhoods are complex, multidimensional ecosystems that are shaped by forces from within and without. For example, although the focus of this chapter is on the neighborhood as a habitat and a niche unto itself, it would be remiss to not mention that larger macroeconomic, social, and political blueprints (1) locate children and families in particular neighborhoods and (2) influence the ascendancy and degradation of those neighborhoods. It is imperative that family health social work practitioners who endeavor to work within neighborhoods recognize how neighborhood contexts and the resources within them are shaped by social, economic, and political structures that are founded on hierarchies of economics, skin color, language, gender, sexuality, ability, and culture. This should be kept in mind as the multidimensional aspects of neighborhood are explored.

Neighborhood can be conceived of as a complex conglomeration that comprises four general categories: social composition, economic composition, social processes, and physical composition/resources. Examples of the elements associated with these categories are listed in Box 12.1.

In considering the four categories in Box 12.1, it is important to differentiate between neighborhood as environment (habitat) and neighborhood as place (niche). For example, the family health social work practitioner, who is most often an "outsider" to a child and

BOX 12.1.
Four general categories of the construct neighborhood.

1. *Social composition*
       Age
       Race/ethnicity
       Nativity
       Residential mobility
       Density of children
       Percent of female headed households
       Percent of elderly and percent of single parents
2. *Economic composition*
       Percent affluent neighbors
       Poverty
       Employment
       Percent white-collar workers
       Percent managerial/professional workers
       Education
       Public housing
       Home ownership
3. *Social processes*
       Organizational participation
       Unsupervised teens
       Neighboring
       Crime
       Value consensus
       Community monitoring
       Social capital/social networks
4. *Physical composition/resources*
       Condition of housing
       Trash/litter
       Graffiti
       Traffic and street conditions
       Playgrounds/parks
       Proximity to employment
       Community centers
       Schools
       Bars
       Libraries
       Abandoned homes
       Vacant lots
       Architecture

Source: Nicotera, in press, pp. 102-103.

family's neighborhood, may view it as a habitat or environment that can be assessed in terms of its structural characteristics which include social composition, economic composition, and physical composition/ resources as described in Box 12.1. This view can lead to what Kemp (2001) calls the outsider's laundry list of problems within the environment and can result in deficit-oriented assessments.

However, it is the third category noted in Box 12.1, social processes, that constitutes neighborhood as a place or niche and provides the potential for a deeper and more strengths-based comprehension of the neighborhood ecosystem. For is it through social processes or the lived experiences of "insiders" that a neighborhood becomes more than its structural characteristics and takes on meaning for the children and families who reside within it? For example, Tuan (cited in Dixon and Durrheim, 2000) notes that

> language becomes the force that binds people to places, it is through language that everyday experiences of self-in-place form and mutate, moreover, it is through language that places themselves are imaginatively constituted in ways that carry implications for who we are (or who we claim to be). (p. 32)

Therefore, to fully comprehend the entity called *neighborhood* with all of its challenges and strengths, it is necessary for the family health social work practitioner to understand the neighborhood as a habitat, a niche, and the transactional processes through which macrosocial, economic, and political blueprints; neighborhood habitats; and neighborhood niches have the capacity to influence and shape one another. The literature review that follows provides the reader with a sense of neighborhood as habitat and niche. Recommended readings listed in part five of the chapter direct interested readers to literature that addresses neighborhood in the context of macrosocial, economic, and political blueprints.

PART TWO: LITERATURE REVIEW FROM THE ADULT'S WORLDVIEW

The literature that examines neighborhood as a factor in the lives of children and families encompasses a variety of disciplines, such as social work, sociology, community psychology, environmental psychology, urban planning, and geography. This multidisciplinary body of literature provides a basis from which to understand the ways in which neighborhoods influence children and families. This review examines research that uncovers the manner in which the social and physical environments of neighborhoods can influence human behavior. It is summarized in terms of the three questions noted at the outset of this chapter. This review, as well as the review in part three of the chapter and their respective summaries, is aimed at increasing the family health social work practitioner's ability to understand the dynamics of neighborhood habitats and niches.

Several researchers provide insight into how the physical and social environment of a neighborhood can influence human behavior. The physical configuration and conditions of the built environment of a neighborhood impact one's experience within it. This is supported by the work of Skejaeveland and Garling (1997), who examined the connection between the built environment and neighboring behavior within neighborhoods. The results of their study indicate that neighboring behavior can be predicted from objective and perceived measures of spaciousness. This study also found that visual appearance, including such items as "upkeep of building property, interior and exterior appearances and the presence of greeneries," predicted neighboring behavior (p. 191).

In addition to neighboring, the physical and social aspects of a neighborhood can also be a factor in residents' sense of safety and assessment of the level of neighborhood problems. For example, Perkins, Meeks, and Taylor (1992) examined how physical incivilities and social incivilities within a neighborhood (Baltimore, Maryland) related to residents' feelings of danger in the locale. Physical incivilities are defined as litter, vandalism, vacant or dilapidated housing, abandoned cars, and unkempt lots. Social incivilities include loitering youths, prostitutes, homeless people, rowdy behavior, drug dealing, and public drunkenness (Perkins, Meeks, and Taylor 1992). The authors found that physical incivilities are linked to resident perceptions of social incivilities and crime. The level of fear and perceptions of neighborhood problems by neighborhood residents plays a role in human behavior, as Coulton's (1996) study indicates. Coulton found that the level of fear in a neighborhood, resulting from violence and drug trafficking, was related to residents' avoidance of it either by moving or by isolating themselves and their children from the neighborhood if they could not afford to move (Coulton, 1996). This study is supported by the work of Sampson and Raudenbush (1999), which provides evidence that neighborhood social disorder (e.g., adults loitering, public drinking, peer groups with signs of gang affiliation) and neighborhood physical disorder (e.g., garbage or litter, empty beer bottles, graffiti) were negatively "moderately strongly correlated with survey measures of collective efficacy ($r = -.49$ for social disorder; $r = -.47$ for physical disorder, $p < .01$)" (p. 623) and that "collective efficacy is the strongest predictor of violent victimization ($B = -.37$, $t = -3.59$, $p < .01$)" (p. 627).

In summary, these studies provide evidence that the physical and social environments of a neighborhood have the potential to influence the behavior of its residents in such a way that the potential for social support and collective action among neighbors is diminished or does not have the chance to blossom when habitats are characterized by physical and social incivilities. This lack of social support or social cohesion can have a great impact on parents as they work to safely and successfully raise their children, and certainly points to an arena for assessment and intervention for family health social work practitioners. In fact, the last two studies reviewed in this section provide evidence of how neighborhood influences parenting behaviors.

Furstenberg (1993) points out that the social characteristics of neighborhood environments can either support or constrain parents' capabilities for helping their children toward "school completion and the attainment of economic security, staying out of trouble with the law, the postponement of childbearing, and avoidance of excessive use of drugs and alcohol" (p. 236). He notes that "family management strategies tied to the community may be no less consequential for children's development than the more direct, proximate controls observed inside the home" (p. 233).

In support of this idea, Furstenberg (1993) draws the following conclusion from his ethnographic study of parents in different Philadelphia, Pennsylvania, neighborhoods. Irrespective of parenting-skill levels, the parents residing in a neighborhood characterized by lack of services for parents and teenagers, the presence of only a few community organizations (all of which were suffering from budget cuts), lack of trust between neighbors, and problems with dangers presented by drug dealers and other street crimes were more likely to function as individuals in parenting their children as opposed to accessing local resources and neighbors for a more collective parenting strategy (Furstenberg, 1993). Parents in this type of neighborhood exemplify an absence of ties to the neighborhood, noting in general that their main goal is to survive there until they can locate a better residence (Furstenberg, 1993). Furstenberg found a minimal level of social integration, meaning that although there was a surface type of familiarity among residents, it was typical for neighbors to not even know the names of residents with whom they had some social interaction. One parent in this neighborhood noted mistrust of her neighbors and "express[ed] misgivings about community institutions. She criticiz[ed] many of her neighbors for being far too permissive with their children and inattentive to the ever-present dangers of drugs and drug-related violence" (Furstenberg, 1993, p. 239). This parent's fifteen-year-old daughter attends school and socializes with friends from outside the neighborhood. The parent also describes why she takes her children to the health clinic outside of the neighborhood. "Now see, the clinic my kids go to, it's all bright and lively. Even if you is sick, you don't be looking like I'm going to die. But that place (referring to the clinic near the Projects) looked like the slaughterhouse" (Furstenberg, 1993, p. 241).

Brodsky's (1996) study, conducted in Washington, DC, found similar results. The mothers in Brodsky's study worked very hard to isolate themselves and their children from the effects of the neighborhoods in which they lived and thus, they were, as Furstenberg would point out, left to "manage on their own" (1993, p. 243). One of the mothers in Brodsky's (1996) study provides an example of this concept when she describes the terrifying experience she and her children had when gunshots went on for an hour one New Year's Eve. This mother noted that even though the whole neighborhood shared the experience, she alone provided her children with the comfort and explanations they required. In reference to handling the incident within her family as opposed to among neighbors, she says:

> I don't go out here, I don't start things with people. I don't bother people. I go home, I close my door, I lock my door, I stay in my house. Don't bother me and I won't bother you. Don't bother my kids, I won't bother you. (Brodsky, 1996, p. 357)

The mothers in Brodsky's (1996) study mirror as well the mistrust in local services that Furstenberg (1993) notes. One of the mothers in

Brodsky's (1996) study reflects this mistrust when she describes how the school responded negatively to her when she spoke up about what she felt was right.

In addition to lack of trust in local resources and social connections with neighbors, "many families in socially disorganized neighborhoods either had few kin living close by or, for one reason or another, had weak ties with relatives" (Furstenberg, 1993, p. 241). "Lillie has no family living close by. Maria's extended kin were all back in Puerto Rico. Ida, one of the parents in North Park, could not rely on her kin because virtually all were involved in drug trade or were addicts themselves" (Furstenberg, 1993, p. 241).

In contrast to the previously noted experiences of parents, Furstenberg (1993) spoke to parents who lived in a different Philadelphia neighborhood that, although troubled by problems with drug dealers and drug-related violence, was characterized by the presence of social cohesion. The parents in this neighborhood, who shared similar backgrounds to the parents in the less socially cohesive neighborhood just described, reported parenting strategies that were less isolating.

Many of the residents grew up in this neighborhood and note the pride they have in the range of local kin networks and friendship ties. As Furstenberg (1993) notes, "All the families that we observed in the Heights [shortened name for this neighborhood] had at least one grandparent living within walking distance and all had other siblings living nearby" (p. 244). In addition to family, neighborhood children are under the watch of other adult residents in the neighborhood. Furstenberg pointed out that the community businesses and institutions were run by local residents who were a visible presence within the neighborhood. One parent in this neighborhood stated, "Somebody's always watching over the kids. Not just my family here. But just people I know on the block, in the neighborhood" (Furstenberg, 1993, p. 246). An example of this watchfulness can be found in Furstenberg's study. When one of the neighborhood children slipped out of his home one night, his mother called a couple of the boy's friends to let him know he had better get home, and he arrived within ten minutes. Furstenberg (1993) points out that even though the mother of this particular child did not exhibit the strongest parenting skills, the "close lateral links within generations allow[ed] parents like [her] to receive invisible or barely visible forms of assistance" (p. 248).

In conjunction with these more informal supports for parenting, this particular neighborhood has strong local resources through which adults participate in the care and guidance of the neighborhood children. For example, an administrator for the local Catholic school lives in the neighborhood, and, in addition to her employment at the school, she runs a crafts class for the neighborhood children in the park. This horizontal tie within the neighborhood became a vertical tie when this same woman's brother-in-law employed his connections with the city to obtain assistance in funding several teen programs in the neighborhood (Furstenberg, 1993).

The main difference between these two neighborhoods, besides the level of social cohesion, is found in the levels of socioeconomic status. Although the parents in the studies were similar in terms of family structure and welfare use, the neighborhood with less social cohesion was in one of the "poorest sections of North Philadelphia . . . whereas [parents in the more socially cohesive neighborhood] live[d] on one of the less desirable blocks of a small, white working-class enclave in South Philadelphia" (Furstenberg, 1993, p. 237). Therefore, poor families benefit from living adjacent to comparatively more affluent working-class neighbors.

Furstenberg's (1993) study included a third neighborhood, which he portrayed as a *transitional neighborhood*. This neighborhood is characterized by the out-migration of working and middle-class families; an increase in residents who are unemployed, single mothers, and welfare recipients; local industries that have been in decline for some years, and the "withdrawal of government funds for local programs and services" (p. 250). Furstenberg (1993) points out that this transition is accompanied by shifts from collective parenting strategies to more isolating individualistic strategies.

Box 12.2 provides a summary of how the research just reviewed informs the three questions noted at the beginning of the chapter. It presents the family health social work practitioner with the elements of neighborhood habitats and niches that have the potential for both positively and negatively affecting the children and families that she or he serves. Box 12.2 suggests the aspects of a neighborhood that can serve as a resource for children and families as well as arenas for intervention.

The first question in Box 12.2 assists in assessment of the habitat or the neighborhood environment. Some of the elements associated

---

BOX 12.2.
Elements of neighborhood habitats and niches that affect
children and families.

1. Who is involved in the ecosystem from the immediate to the extended environment and who makes up the habitat? (When it comes to the neighborhood, one can add to this question by also including, "What" is in the habitat?)	Kin Neighbors Business owners Drug dealers Drunks Youths Prostitutes School personnel Homeless people Role models	Schools Businesses Community Orgs. Parks Vacant buildings Litter Fences Sidewalks Clinics Dilapidated homes
2. What kinds of niches do individuals and families occupy? How do they perceive themselves and their niches?	Perceptions of: Spaciousness Crimes Hazards Greeneries Upkeep of homes	Perceptions of: Insiders Outsiders Level of trust Quality of resources Level of safety
3. How have these niches positively and negatively affected the individuals and families in relation to other people and institutions in that environment?	Neighboring Social interactions Collective efficacy Isolation Funding	Mobility patterns Parenting strategy Health of busineses Level of trust

---

with this question can be assessed visually by the family health social work practitioner, whereas others, such as kin, neighbors, and role models, can be discovered in conversation with neighborhood residents. Niches (the elements associated with questions 2 and 3) are best assessed through conversation with neighborhood residents, business owners, and employees of neighborhood resources.

Assessment of both the habitat and niche are imperative because the family health social work practitioner may note several resources available at the habitat level, for example, a community center and a neighborhood park, that residents do not view as resources because of perceptions of lack of quality or levels of drug dealing on the corner adjacent to the resource. Therefore, assessments of habitat need to be grounded in assessments of niche, which can occur only via conversations with neighborhood residents.

Knowledge gleaned from thorough assessments of habitats and niches should lead to the development of appropriate interventions. For example, when vacant lots, dilapidated homes, and public drunkenness create fear and lack of trust among neighborhood residents, the family health social work practitioner may work on a macrolevel that engages landlords, homeowners, and local police to increase attention and care of the neighborhood. Interventions such as these require knowledge of the macro social, economic, and political blueprints that shape and have shaped the neighborhood habitat. For example, in many neighborhoods, dilapidated housing and levels of public drunkenness persist because of the negative perceptions due to racism and classism of landlords and local police who do not reside in the neighborhood. Interventions for such cases are more complex and require the family health social work practitioner to educate distal landlords and police as well as work with residents in self-advocacy.

Interventions may also occur at a microlevel to influence an increase in social connections when neighborhood residents report self-imposed isolation and lack of trust in other neighborhood residents. Knowledge about how human behaviors and perceptions of niche are influenced by the conditions of the neighborhood habitat is key to the development of appropriate interventions. For example, the family health social work practitioner who endeavors to increase collective-parenting strategies needs to be cognizant of the reasons why, as described in the literature, such strategies do not already exist in the neighborhood.

Finally, recognition of the reciprocal relationship between habitat and niche allows the practitioner to consider intervention at either the macro- or microlevel as a means for creating change. For example, an intervention at the macrolevel, such as the one just discussed, has the potential to change the habitat such that families' perceptions of the niche allow them to move from individualistic parenting strategies to more collective ones. On the other hand, intervention at the microlevel to increase social connections and trust among neighborhood residents has the potential to increase social cohesion and in turn create the basis for collective efficacy that can lead to changes in the neighborhood habitat or environment.

PART THREE: LITERATURE REVIEW FROM THE CHILD'S WORLDVIEW

The research studies just reviewed clearly demonstrate the influence of the social and physical environment of the neighborhood ecosystem on human behavior, and, in particular, on neighboring behavior, collective efficacy, and strategies of parenting. This section of the chapter is concerned with how our understanding of the neighborhood ecosystem can be informed by the voices of children. Curiously, although children are an integral part of families as well as the target population of much of social work practice and research, their perceptions and experiences have occupied a peripheral place in these endeavors. With few exceptions (e.g., Bryant, 1985; Burton and Price-Spratlen, 1999; Hart, 1979; Moore, 1986; Nicotera, 2003; Sutton, 1992), researchers of neighborhood habitats and niches have presumed knowledge of children's experiences based on the perceptions of the adults around them, on structural and demographic information about their families, and the neighborhoods in which they reside. In addition, in the arena of social work practice, the views of children are often considered to be less credible than those of the adult authorities in their lives. However, the family health social work practice model, which notes both empowerment and understanding of how the client constructs her or his reality as some of the important intervention skills for the practitioner (Yuen, 2003), is in a position to give voice to children. The studies reviewed here illuminate the child's perspective on neighborhood. They also suggest potential sites for assessment and intervention by the family health social work practitioner as he or she explores the neighborhood as a resource for the children and families with whom he or she works.

One of the more recent studies on child-neighborhood interactions (Lewis and Osofsky, 1997) reports on children's drawings about their neighborhoods in a moderately sized, southern (U.S.) city. Children in the study were between the ages of eight and twelve, and all of them were African Americans who resided in low-income neighborhoods, some of which were known for high rates of violence. Children were asked to draw two pictures, one of their neighborhood and the second of what goes on in their neighborhood. In general, 9 percent of the children included depictions of violence in response to the general question "draw a picture of your neighborhood," and more than 60 percent of the children drew pictures that portrayed violence when drawing in response to the question, "What goes on in your neighborhood?" (Lewis and Osofsky, 1997).

The researchers defined violence in the drawings as "an act or behavior that causes damage or injury, or human figures engaged in verbal threats or activity labeled as fighting, hitting, or someone starting a fire or robbery" (Lewis and Osofsky, 1997, p. 283). One eight-year-old boy drew a picture that portrayed one girl shooting another, a box shape labeled drugs, and a person in a car. The child wrote, "A girl shot a other girl" on the picture (Lewis and Osofsky, 1997, p. 284). Another child (age and gender not noted) drew a picture titled "Killing/Drugs" that depicts one person shooting another. A third picture showed a person labeled "Lady" saying, "Don't cry run" (Lewis and Osofsky, 1997, p. 287). There are figures that are labeled: bad man, good man, gangster, police, ambulance, Jeff, and Linda (who are crying). The figures labeled "bad man" and "gangster" are holding or shooting guns. None of the other figures are holding or shooting weapons. In contrast to these drawings, the authors present pictures by children that do not contain violence, even though they were drawn in response to the question of what happens in their neighborhood. These contain children playing and smiling figures with words such as "love" written on them.

In summary, the children's drawings are enlightening, and one can use them to speculate on children's neighborhood experiences; however, one cannot do much beyond speculation without some other kind of information from the children, whether it is about their pictures directly or about their neighborhoods in general. Hence, it is difficult to comprehend, from drawings alone, how neighborhood environments may influence the meanings that children make for themselves and the world around them, and, in turn, how neighborhoods may be useful as a resource in family health social work practice. The chapter turns now to studies that provide more direct details from children about their neighborhoods.

One such study, completed in a mid-sized city in the Netherlands, asked children about places they liked and disliked in their neighborhoods, and why (van Andel, 1990). The sample consisted of 140 children between the ages of six and twelve who lived in three different neighborhoods. The three neighborhoods are described in terms of physical layout but not in terms of socioeconomic or demographic information. The study asked children about places they thought were attractive, boring, or dangerous.

Children in all three neighborhoods were most likely to mention places they liked, which tended to include parks or other natural, green areas. The propensity for children to note places such as these coincided with whether or not such areas existed within their neighborhoods. The reasons that children gave for liking any specific area within their neighborhood were that it allowed them to (1) participate in some activity, such as riding bikes or playing soccer; (2) have access to natural items such as trees or simply wide open space; and (3) be in the company of other children (van Andel, 1990).

Children in this study were less likely to note boring areas within their neighborhoods, and nearly half of the areas labeled boring were playgrounds and streets. The reasons that children gave for the boring nature of these areas were: (1) too much traffic, (2) obstacles that prevented them from playing, (3) litter or other messes, and (4) other children who were mean. As for places children viewed as dangerous, the street was most often mentioned. The danger in the streets was noted to be due to the quantity of cars and the speed at which they traveled. Children noted the potential for being involved in an accident due to the vehicles in the street. This sense of danger is dramatically different from the depictions in the children's drawings noted in Lewis and Osofsky's (1997) study with children in low-income neighborhoods in the United States.

Another study in which children were queried about their neighborhoods was conducted by Schiavo (1988), who worked with fifty-nine children between the ages of eight and eighteen who attended public schools and resided in a middle-class suburban area about fifteen miles outside Boston, Massachusetts. Children were asked to evaluate their neighborhood in terms of its characteristics and the activities that took place in it. In addition, children were given a camera in order to take up to twenty-four photographs of "any place [inside or outside] in the home or neighborhood that's important to you, any place you care about" (Schiavo, 1988, p. 5). Participants were then interviewed about the photos they took. Although the children photographed people, animals, and physical places, Schiavo reports on only the photos that involved physical places.

When queried about what they liked the best about the neighborhood, children noted: (1) features that allowed for activities such as bike riding or playing and (2) positive social relationships with "friends and/or among neighbors" (Schiavo, 1988, p. 5). The characteristics children disliked within the neighborhood were busy streets, yard sizes, or the absence of children within their age group. In contrast, the main feature of the neighborhood that participants felt was positive for adolescents was its proximity to "highways to get to movies and shopping areas" (Schiavo, 1988, p. 5).

The participants' photographs of places they deemed important include "nature sites, street/cul-de-sac, elementary school, friend's house, athletic facilities, store/business, public building (library) and neighbors' homes" (Schiavo, 1988, p. 7). It is notable that as the participants reached older adolescence they became less place dependent, or they mentioned diminished linkages to the neighborhood of residence for activities and social relations. Instead they were more aligned with neighborhoods of sociability or places where they spent time among peers. This is important information for the family health social work practitioner who serves families with teenagers. In such cases, practitioners will want to assess the adolescent's neighborhood of residence as well as her or his neighborhood of sociability. Another form of research in which children talk about their residential locations results in more open-ended depictions of the neighborhood environments.

Moore (1986) worked with children in the London area to learn about: "their specific interactions with their surroundings . . . [Moore's] starting point in understanding the relationship between play, place, and child development, was to find out what children actually did, where, when, with what, with whom—when not in class or at home engaged in routine chores" (Moore, 1986, p, xvii). The participants in the study were ninety-six children ages nine to twelve who lived in three different "city" neighborhoods. All of the children completed a drawing in response to the request to draw a "map or drawing of all of your favorite places—where you go after school or at weekends, including summer—around your home, in the neighbourhood where you live" (Moore, 1986, p. 268). Each child also participated in a fifteen- to twenty-minute interview. In addition, about one-quarter of the children participated in "field trips" in which they acted as experts who took the researcher on a trip around the territory of their neighborhoods (Moore, 1986).

Since the data that can be gleaned from children's drawings have already been noted, the findings from Moore's field trips with the children will be discussed here. One child noted a shed behind her home in which she played. "She and her best friend Lesley led me [Moore] down some outdoor steps to a door below their garage. A small sign proclaimed Hair Bear Mansion. They said the name came from a TV show" (Moore, 1986, p. 84). Moore goes on to describe the interior of this play space, which included a set of posted rules and announcements for contests such as who could procure the best piece of material for the creation of a costume. One of the girls had a written a play, and the costumes would be used for that. Also, the date of the founding of the club was posted on a wall, and the girls had a suggestion box. Evidence of suggestions was noted from a list on the wall (Moore, 1986).

Another child took Moore on a field trip to another indoor "child-owned" space. This space was in an abandoned building that had burned. The child pointed out how he and a friend had swept the floor and created furniture from old boards and bricks. Another child showed Moore an abandoned house in which she and her friends played. The child told Moore that people said the house was haunted, and that she did not believe in ghosts but that "there could be nasty men there"; therefore she would not go in by herself (Moore, 1986, p. 187). She described a game, called "murder in the dark," that she and her peers played inside the house, and also how they looked for ladybirds and picked blackberries in the garden behind the house. There are many other aspects of children's neighborhood experiences explored by Moore, but these few anecdotes provide a perspective on neighborhood environments that is unique to children.

The perspectives noted here, from Moore's (1986) study, provide some intimate details about the kinds of adventures children have within their neighborhoods. The next two studies represent other views of neighborhoods from the child's perspective. Burton and Price-Spratlen (1999) report data from a five-year ethnographic study conducted in a northeastern (U.S.) city where they learned about "community and family beliefs concerning the definitions of neighborhood, neighborhood processes, and the life-course development of urban African American children, teens, and adults" (p. 83). Some of the quotes from children in this study (1) define neighborhood, (2) note the multiple neighborhoods negotiated by children, and (3) describe the interactive influence of neighborhood on child and child on neighborhood.

Burton and Price-Spratlen (1999) note the differences between adult and child definitions of neighborhood boundaries. In fact, in 56 percent of the cases in their study, the children and adolescents defined the boundaries of the neighborhood in a manner that greatly contrasted the boundaries noted by the adults. One eight-year-old boy said,

> Well, my neighborhood is where my best friends live. Eric lives on the corner of Anderson, Devon lives in the middle of the block on Tyree Street, and Jason lives at the end of the street on Beacon . . . my neighborhood doesn't go past those streets either way. That's my neighborhood. (Burton and Price-Spratlen, 1999, p. 85)

This child's mother defined the boundaries of his (the child's) neighborhood to include an area of five blocks in one direction and eight blocks in another because it was the parameters within which the child could travel on foot without her and be safe (Burton and Price-Spratlen, 1999).

Another child, an eleven-year-old boy, provides an example of the multiple neighborhoods a child may need to negotiate. He states,

> Lady, I think you're pretty smart, so let me tell you how it is. When I go to my momma's I have to be a bad ass or I will get beat up. So if you see me over there, I look like that. But when I'm with Nana (grandmother) I'm another way 'cause the kids over there don't fight that much so I don't have to swell up (act like he's tough). (Burton and Price-Spratlen, 1999, p. 87)

Finally, a twelve-year-old boy in their sample suggests the way in which the neighborhood can influence residents and vice versa. He says,

> My neighborhood so bad is cause some of the young bloods here is bad. Just cause it's all junky round here don't mean peo-

ple in it got to be junky on the inside. If young brothers round here get together, we could make it a good place. Some my friends don't know that it be bad here cause they be bad not cause the neighborhood make them bad. (Burton and Price-Spratlen, 1999, p. 88)

Nicotera (2003) conducted the final study reviewed in this section. It involved fifty-nine fourth- and fifth-grade children who responded to several different open-ended writing activities in which they were queried about their neighborhoods (thirty census tracts) and their neighbors in the greater Seattle area of Washington State. The sample of children consisted of a diverse group of boys (48 percent) and girls (52 percent) representing Euro-Americans (42.4 percent), Asians and Pacific Islanders (18.6 percent), Native Americans (15.2 percent), Mexican Americans (8.5 percent), Hispanic children of color (6.8 percent), African Americans (5.1 percent), Hispanic whites (1.7 percent), and Africans (1.7 percent).

Results demonstrate that the neighborhood niches have a great capacity to support and challenge children. The difference between this study and those reviewed thus far is that the results provide information about how children actually interact with their neighbors in ways that promote the development of certain competencies. It also indicates that neighbors provide children with both tangible and intangible support. In addition, the results point to the challenges faced by children as they perceive their neighborhood niches (Nicotera, 2003).

The niches, as perceived by the children, support them in the development of a number of competencies, including physicality, cognition, social-emotional capacity, nurturing abilities, and skills for independence. These competencies were gained via social interaction with neighbors (Nicotera, 2003). For example, some of the children noted that they had increased their skills in basketball, swimming, jumping rope, and roller skating because of the assistance they received from neighbors. Others mentioned how neighbors had helped them with homework and school projects. Aside from these more tangible competencies, children wrote about how neighbors supported their development of social-emotional skills and skills for independence. For example, one child wrote, "Dear J. You have taught me how to face my fears," and another wrote, "Dear Mr. B. These are some of the things I have learned from you. 1. If you give someone something they will give me something back, 2. You should be nice" (Nicotera,

2003, p. 186). The children often reported that they had gained competence on several levels through their interactions with one neighbor. For example, a child noted, "Dear S. You have taught me how to be a gentleman. And you have taught me manners. You have taught me how to use a computer and how to play games. You have also taught me how to save money and put it in a safe place" (Nicotera, 2003, p. 187). Finally, among other competencies, the children in this study indicated that they were acquiring the ability to nurture others as a result of their relationships with neighbors. For example, one child wrote about a neighbor who has helped her learn about taking care of a baby and the things that make a baby happy. The child indicates that this has made her a more confident babysitter (Nicotera, 2003).

In addition to the development of competence, the children in this study indicated that neighbors played important roles in providing social supports. For example, one child mentioned a neighbor who babysits her and also drives her to school, and another wrote about a neighbor who takes her to the library. Finally, one child wrote, "You have helped me by telling me lots of different advice for when I grow up. . . . You helped me by being kind to me" (Nicotera, 2003, p. 239). The neighborhoods in which the children in this sample reside also provide them with opportunities to "hang out" with friends, buy things at the store, go to the library, ride bikes, build forts, and to be inside their own or a friend's house to watch TV or play video games.

The experiences and perceptions of the children in this study were not always positive. They mentioned some of the challenges they faced in their neighborhoods. Many of these challenges were discovered as a result of asking the children to describe places they did not like in their neighborhoods. The children shared many emotions as they wrote about the places in their neighborhoods that they disliked. Some noted more benign feelings such as being bored or feeling crowded, and others wrote about scary and dangerous people or places, broken glass and other litter, feeling lonely, and about people who ranged from the "mean lady across the street" to the mean neighbor who "shot my dog and stole my 'trading cards'" (Nicotera, 2003, p. 231). For example, one child wrote this about a convenience store: "I do not like because it attracts drunks, smokers, and people who sell drugs" (Nicotera, 2003, p. 197). Another child wrote about the stairs at an apartment building, "The stairs are cracked and somebody could fall and break you leg," and someone else wrote "Thair [there] is no neighbor I like. One shot my dog. The other moved away" (Nicotera, 2003, pp. 223, 231).

Thus, the children in this study present the neighborhood as both a niche that supports the development of important life skills and a place that confronts them with challenges. Some of the challenges and concerns reported by this sample are similar to those found in the other studies reviewed here. However, the social supports as perceived by the children in this study (Nicotera 2003) are not present in the other studies in which children are respondents.

Regardless, all of the studies reviewed here suggest that neighborhoods have the potential to serve as a resource for children and families. Family health social work practitioners are in a position to harness and develop those resources as means for assisting the children and families they serve. An exploration of how this can be accomplished considers these studies based on Yuen's (2003) questions aimed at assisting the family health social work practitioner in increasing her or his capacity to understand an ecosystem: (1) who and what makes up the neighborhood habitat, (2) what kinds of niches do children and families perceive, and (3) how have these niches positively and negatively affected the children and families in relation to other people and institutions in the neighborhood? (See Box 12.3.)

A quick comparison between Box 12.2 in part three of this chapter and Box 12.3 demonstrates the different realities that adults and children construct within a neighborhood ecosystem. The family health social work practitioner who endeavors to use the neighborhood as a resource for her or his work with children and families would be well advised to consider the voices of both the children and adults in the family. Assessment strategies with children require methods beyond conversation. The literature reviewed in this chapter suggests several strategies for the assessment of a child's neighborhood habitat and niche. These include: children's drawings of what happens in one's neighborhood, drawing a map of one's favorite places in the neighborhood, child-directed photographs of the neighborhood, child-led tours of the neighborhood, and written or oral responses to queries about the child's neighborhood and neighbors.

Bryant (1985) offers an excellent tool to structure a child-led tour of a neighborhood that is titled "The Neighborhood Walk." This technique involves fifteen questions posed to the child during the walk

---

BOX 12.3
Questions and answers concerning
how to understand an ecosystem.

1. Who is involved in the ecosystem from the immediate to the extended environment and who makes up the habitat? (When it comes to the neighborhood one can add to this question by also including, "What" is in the habitat?)

Bad man
Good man
One girl shot
    another
Gangster
Police
Ambulance
Children
Friend's house
Library
Club house
Helpful neighbors

Parks
Playgrounds
Streets
Traffic
Litter
Trees
Animals
Good places
    to play
School
Stores/
    businesses
Drugs and
    dealers

2. What kinds of niches do individuals and families occupy? How do they perceive themselves and their niches?

Perception of:
Violence
Love
Boring
Dangerous
Attractive
Mean people
Junky
Easy access out

Perception of:
Too much
    traffic
Mean children
No kids my age
Best friend
Child-owned
    space
Fear
Nice and clean
Self

3. How have these niches positively and negatively affected the individuals and families in relation to other people and institutions in that environment?

Friends to play
    with
Fear of violence
Fun activities
Competence
Support

One setting
    "bad ass"
another "I'm
    not"
Limitations
Opportunities

---

around the neighborhood and twenty-one questions to be completed after the walk. Bryant used this tool successfully with children in first, second, fourth, and fifth grade. The questions provide information about a variety of elements in the child's neighborhood world, including where the child plays with peers, places he or she goes to be alone, neighbors he or she visits, neighborhood animals or pets with whom he or she associates, and friendships.

Nicotera (2003) provides examples of questions that can be utilized to gather information about a child's perceptions of her or his neighborhood habitat and niche, including neighbors who may serve as important social supports. This series of questions can be posed as an oral activity between the family health social work practitioner and one child, or as written exercises for larger groups of children. They have been utilized successfully with fourth- and fifth-grade students. These questions involve asking children to

1. discuss places in their neighborhoods they like and do not like and to explain why,
2. describe what they would change in their neighborhood if they were in charge and how that would make the neighborhood different from its current state,
3. think about a neighbor they like and describe why they like that neighbor and some of the things that neighbor does, and
4. describe the things a neighbor they like does for them and things they have learned from that neighbor.

Assessment tools such as those described here provide the family health social work practitioner with the child's-eye view of her or his neighborhood experiences that points to areas of support and sites of intervention at both micro- and macrolevels. For example, at the microlevel it is clear that children will benefit from talking and playing about the stressful events they witness in their neighborhoods. Also, neighbors identified by children as social support can play a role in supporting this talk and play. In addition, they can be harnessed as resources to support collective-parenting strategies within a neighborhood.

At the macrolevel, children of all ages have the capacity to name what needs to be changed in their neighborhoods and to participate in creating that change (Hart, 1997). In fact, the neighborhood characteristics children would like to change are often similar to those that adults would want to change. For example, when queried about what they would change if they were in charge of their neighborhoods, some of the things children mentioned are (1) creating a park in which one can hear the birds sing, (2) reducing traffic and installing stoplights to control traffic, (3) getting rid of "punks" who smoke and do drugs, and (4) creating safe places to play (Nicotera, in press). Clearly, these types of changes require some level of neighborhood social cohesion and collective efficacy, both of which, as the literature states, are influenced by neighborhood physical and social conditions. The next part of this chapter offers a case study of a child's neighborhood habitat and niche as a means for further exploring the role of neighborhood in family health social work practice.

PART FOUR: CASE STUDY AND APPLICATION

This part of the chapter presents a case study of a child and family within a neighborhood habitat and niche. After reading the case study, the reader is invited to share in an application of the family health social work practice model as a means to assess and consider intervention to ameliorate the presenting problem.

Case Study

Marta is an eleven-year-old Mexican-American girl in the fifth grade. She is the only child of two working parents. Her mother is a librarian, and her father is an engineer. She has excellent scholastic skills and gets along well with her teachers and peers at school. Therefore, it is a surprise when her parents contact you, the school social worker, and share the following concerns: (1) she does not play with any peers when she is at home, (2) she prefers to stay in her room watching TV and listening to music, and (3) when her parents banned TV and music on the weekends in an effort to force her to play outside, she became sullen and lethargic.

Her parents are worried that Marta is depressed and wonder if her behavior could be signs of early adolescent rebellion. They explain that she did not behave this way before they relocated to the new neighborhood about a year and a half ago. They report that when they ask her about her behavior, Marta's only response is to say she wants to stay at home where she feels safe. Her parents tell you that they are not sure why she feels this way because the new neighborhood seems so nice and peaceful to them. In fact, they tell you that they moved to this neighborhood because they felt it was safer than where they had lived previously. When you ask if Marta has also changed schools since the move, they tell you that she has been in the same school since kindergarten.

Application: Assessment Phase

The family health social work practice model suggests that you, the social worker, consider this case from several different theoretical viewpoints that include the following: ecological perspectives, systems theory, social constructionism and diversity, and developmental and family theories. Marta's positive behavior and progress at school indicate that she is on track in terms of her individual life course. Your interactions with her parents and initial assessment indicate that the family is functioning well as an open system. Your assessment of Marta as a person within her school habitat and niche indicate an array of strengths and healthy psychological and social functioning within that environment.

In order to explore what might be the source of the behaviors or coping activities that concern Marta's parents, you examine the ecological factors in her life, including her neighborhood habitat (environment) and niche (the meaning or social construction she has attached to the neighborhood as a place). Gaining an understanding of how Marta fits into her new neighborhood is central to your exploration, as that seems to be the site of her difficulties. In essence, you will pose the three questions that have been employed to examine the literature reviewed in parts two and three of this chapter:

1. Who and what makes up Marta's neighborhood habitat?
2. What kind of niche(s) does Marta occupy in her neighborhood? How does she perceive that niche(s) and herself within it (them)?
3. How has that niche(s) positively and negatively affected her and her family?

While Marta's parents have indicated their general view of their neighborhood, after you have explored these questions with Marta, you will want to include her parents in a family discussion of the neighborhood habitat and niche.

There are several ways in which to assess Marta's neighborhood habitat and respond to question one. You can learn about the structural aspects of the neighborhood by obtaining Marta's home address and gathering information about the census tract and/or block group in which she and her parents reside. The census tract represents a larger geographical area than the census block group. (Specific guidelines for accessing census information are provided in the learning exercises in part five of this chapter.) Keep in mind that the literature has demonstrated that the census data provide only a cursory examination of habitat which may or may not be representative of the content and boundaries of Marta's perceived neighborhood. Nevertheless, this information provides a starting point in assessing the neighborhood habitat for levels of income, education, residential stability, and cultural diversity.

In Marta's case, you find that the census data indicate that the population of her "neighborhood" has solid middle-class base with a small percentage (20 percent) of families in upper-middle-class range and an even smaller percentage (16 percent) who live on incomes that are below the poverty line. The rate of unemployment in Marta's neighborhood is only 4.5 percent. These percentages suggest that the neighborhood area has the economic base to support commercial sites and community services. Further examination of Marta's block group within the census tract indicates that she and her family live in a middle-class neighborhood that is bordered by the small percentage of upper-middle-income families who reside in the block group to the east, and the small percentage of families living below the poverty line to the west.

You also learn that about 36 percent of the neighborhood population in the census tract are recent (past five years or so) immigrants, and that in general the census tract is populated by people who had immigrated to the United States at some point in their lifetimes. In addition, the census-tract data indicate that the neighborhood may be in transition since only about 37 percent of the families who live in the neighborhood have been there continuously for the past five years. From this you conjecture that Marta's neighborhood habitat may be in transition, but that it appears to have the capacity to welcome new families as they immigrate to the United States. In effect, the census data would indicate that the tract functions as an open ecosystem. However, you will gain a better sense of this only by grounding your assessment of neighborhood habitat in an assessment of neighborhood as it is perceived or constructed as a niche by residents.

In addition, since the census data do not describe the presence or absence of neighborhood resources such as community centers, parks, libraries, churches, and shops, you will want to ask Marta and her parents about the presence of those in or nearby to their neighborhood. In conjunction, you will want to consider how neighborhood resources have been influenced either positively or negatively by larger economic, social, and political blueprints. This can be accomplished by (1) gathering information about the level of funding and maintenance provided for the resources, (2) cultural and language similarities and/or differences between neighborhood residents and employees/owners of community resources, (3) learning about neighborhood resident involvement with civic organizations that have an influence on the neighborhood, and (4) perceptions of the neighborhood as it is described in news stories and other media.

Another method for learning about Marta's neighborhood habitat is to take a "windshield" survey by driving through on your own and observing the physical environment. You would observe for neighborhood elements such as those identified adjacent to question one in Boxes 12.2 and 12.3 that were presented earlier in this chapter. You will want to remember what the literature suggests about how the presence or absence of these elements might influence parenting behaviors, social cohesion, and collective efficacy. Finally, if Marta and her parents are willing, you could take a "neighborhood walk" (Bryant, 1985) with Marta to discover more about her neighborhood habitat as well as to discover how she perceives her neighborhood as a niche. However, preliminary assessment of Marta's neighborhood niche will help you to decide if the neighborhood is implicated as a true concern that would warrant this more involved activity.

Assessment of Marta's neighborhood niche could occur prior to, simultaneous to, or after some assessment of the neighborhood habitat. Depending on the child, you could choose to ask her to draw, write, or talk about her neighborhood. Several questions that can be utilized in this assessment were presented in part three of this chapter. The reader will recall that the research suggests that asking a child "what goes on in their neighborhood" renders different responses than simply asking them to tell you about their neighborhood. In addition, it is important to pose questions that have the potential to illuminate strengths, such as those suggested by Nicotera (2003) and presented in part three of this chapter. This part of your assessment uncovers that Marta does indeed have some fears about her neighborhood. The only place she likes, in fact, is her home and especially her room where she passes the time watching TV, listening to music, and doing her homework. She perceives herself as safe and comfortable there. You find out that the main place in her neighborhood that she dislikes is the park at the end of her block. She describes it as in the woods, dark and scary, lonely because no kids go there, and she says the only people she's ever seen near the park are homeless or older kids "hanging out." Marta tells you that in her old neighborhood the way she met friends was by playing in the park, but that doesn't work here in her new locale. When you ask about neighbors she tells you that she thinks there are no other kids her age in the neighborhood and that, as far as she knows, there are no kids at her school who live near her. She also indicates that she has not met any adults in her neighborhood. At this point, you may want to further assess Marta's neighborhood by taking a "neighborhood walk" with her (Bryant, 1985).

Application: Intervention Phase

Now that you have gathered some data on Marta's neighborhood as both a habitat and niche, you are ready for a family discussion in which Marta shares her perceptions with her parents so that you can join the family in deciding on the best manner in which to intervene. Although any level of intervention would be followed at the discretion of Marta and her parents, several ideas for intervention are suggested here as examples. At the microlevel, Marta and her parents might decide: (1) to make some social contacts with their neighbors through which Marta may learn of neighborhood peers, (2) to visit the park as a family and talk with Marta about what she sees and has seen there, and/or (3) to increase Marta's social knowledge by learning in an age-appropriate way about homelessness and the systemic causes of homelessness. In addition, since Marta is troubled by the "older kids" and will soon approach adolescence, it might be useful for her parents to start talking with her about the more grown-up choices she will need to be prepared for in her near future.

At the mezzolevel, Marta and her parents might decide to join with you in discovering how other children and parents in the neighborhood feel about the park, and, as a result, a group of families might decide to work with you or on their own on a macrolevel to foster changes in the park that would make it more amenable to children. At the community or macrolevel it would be key to help neighborhood families discuss how their influence as part of the neighborhood ecosystem may create a change in the park that imposes further burden for the homeless people there. The family health social work practice model would support this consideration of how a change to benefit one part of the neighborhood ecosystem could result in a problem for some other part of the system. Finally, at the macrolevel, the neighborhood community may decide to consider the development of activities for the "older kids" hanging out at the park.

PART FIVE: CONCLUSION, LEARNING EXERCISES, AND RECOMMENDED READINGS

In conclusion, the research indicates that neighborhoods do hold both resources and challenges for children and families. Exploring the neighborhood as a habitat and niche coincides with the family health social work practice model's emphasis on holistic wellness. Understanding the dynamics of the neighborhood ecosystems of children and families will lead the family health social work practitioner to more thorough assessments and appropriate interventions. For example, in the case example of Marta and her family, lack of recognition of how Marta's behavior and coping were influenced by her neighborhood residence could lead to inaccurate assessments of clinical depression and/or adolescent rebellion and result in interventions aimed at the wrong target.

The following learning exercises are intended to assist the family health social work practitioner increase his or her ability to consider the neighborhood entity as a focus of assessment and intervention. The recommended readings provide the practitioner with resources for understanding the macro blueprints that influence neighborhood environments. Beyond readings, the practitioner is encouraged to seek out and read the sources that have been cited in this chapter.

Learning Exercises

Accessing Census Data

Use the Internet and go the U.S. Government Census Web site (www.census.gov). When you get to that web page, click on (1) Census 2000, (2) Summary File 3, (3) access to all tables and maps in American FactFinder, and (4) Census 2000 Summary File 3: Detailed Tables. At the top of that page choose "address search." Now type in your home address and hit enter. This will find the census tract and block group number in which you live. Select the geography area you want (tract and block group is most useful) and click on Add and then Next. You should now see a table with a list of census variables. Choose those you want by clicking on each and then on Add, and you will see them appear in the table below. When you have chosen the variables that interest you and added them, click on Show Result. You will see the data that are associated with the variables you chose. If you want to find out the percentages associated with any of these variables, follow this formula: Divide the number associated with the variable that interests you by the total Population listed in the same table. Now multiple that number by 100 and you can find the percentage. You can use this same exercise to learn about the habitat of the children and families with whom you work.

Assessing Neighborhood Habitat

Take a walk through the neighborhood in which you live or through the neighborhood where your social work practice site is located and respond to the following questions. Take notes on each question.

1. Do you observe signs of litter, vandalism, vacant housing, dilapidated housing, abandoned cars, unkempt lots?
2. Do you observe signs of public drunkenness, drug dealing, homelessness?
3. Do you observe overly manicured vacant yards, dwellings with window shades closed, dwellings without front porches, specialized nameplates and number plates on dwellings or mailboxes?
4. Do you observe signs of residents in conversation with one another, children at play, children and adults interacting?
5. What types of dwellings do you observe? For example, apartment buildings (low-rise, high-rise), multifamily dwellings, single-family dwellings.
6. What types of businesses, if any, do you observe? For example, laundromats, banks, grocers, schools, community centers, churches.
7. What types of green spaces do you observe? Are there any built-in features in them? What are they? How are they being

utilized and by what ages? What kind of streets and traffic are nearby the green spaces?

8. How busy are the streets? How fast does traffic move on them? What types of vehicles are driving on them?
9. Do you observe any sidewalks? What kinds of activities, if any, do you observe on the sidewalks?
10. How far apart are dwellings and other buildings in the locale? Are they easily visible from the street and/or sidewalk? Are there any visual barriers, such as privacy fences or hedges between dwellings?

After you have completed this, make a grid of the strengths and challenges of the neighborhood habitat in which you live or practice. Now think about what kinds of messages are communicated by the habitat you have just observed, for example, is it a welcoming environment, a threatening environment? These kinds of considerations lead you to the construction of the neighborhood as place or niche, that is, what kinds of meaning are drawn from this habitat? If you observed the neighborhood that is the site of your social work practice, what does it communicate to the people you serve?

Assessing the Child's-Eye View of the Neighborhood Niche

Engage a child you know in a discussion about her or his neighborhood by asking the following questions. After this discussion, make notes about how the child constructs her or his neighborhood niche. Is the niche constructed in such a way that it supports the child's growth, and why? Is the niche constructed in a way that does not support the child's niche, and why? Use these questions:

1. Tell me about your neighborhood.
2. Tell me about what goes on in your neighborhood.
3. Where do you play, how far from your home is it, how do you get there?
4. Do you go shopping for food with your mom/dad? How do you get there?
5. Where do you go to school, how far from your home is it, how do you get there?

6. Where do your friends live, how far from your home are they, how do you get there?
7. Tell me about a favorite place in your neighborhood. Why is it your favorite place? How often do you get to go there? Does your mom or dad know about this place?
8. Tell me about a place you don't like in your neighborhood. Why is it a place you don't like? Do you ever go there? Does your mom or dad know about this place?
9. Do you know other children in your neighborhood? Do you play with them? What do you do for fun?
10. Do you know adults in your neighborhood, besides the grown ups who live with you? Do you spend any time with them? What do you do when you spend time with them?
11. Tell me about the places you are allowed to go all by yourself in your neighborhood? Tell me about the places you are not allowed to go by yourself in your neighborhood?

Recommended Readings for Understanding the Macro Blueprints That Influence Neighborhood Environments

Kozal, J. (1996) *Amazing grace: The lives of children and the conscience of a nation.* New York: First Harper Perennial.

Medoff, P. and Sklar, H. (1994). *Streets of hope: The fall and rise of an urban neighborhood.* Boston: South End Press.

Sampson, R. and Wilson, W.J. (1995). Toward a theory of race, crime, and urban inequality. In J. Hagan and R. Peterson. (Eds.), *Crime and inequality* (pp. 37-56). Stanford, CA: Stanford University Press.

Sutton, S. (1996). *Weaving a tapestry of resistance: The places, power, and poetry of a sustainable society.* London: Bergin and Garvey.

Wilson. W.J. (1987). *The truly disadvantaged: The inner city, the underclass, and public policy.* Chicago: University of Chicago Press.

Wilson, W.J. (1995). Jobless ghettos and the social outcomes of youngsters. In P. Moen, G. Elder, and K. Luscher, (Eds.), *Examining lives in context: Perspective on the ecology of human development* (pp. 527-543). Washington, DC: American Psychological Association.

Wilson, W.J. (1996). *When work disappears: The world of the new urban poor.* New York: Knopf.

REFERENCES

Brodsky, A. (1996). Resilient single mothers in risky neighborhoods: Negative psychological sense of community. *Journal of Community Psychology, 24*(4), 347-363.

Bryant, L. (1985). The neighborhood walk: Sources of support in middle childhood. *Monographs for the Society of Child Development, 50*(3). Serial No. 210, 118 pps.

Burton, L. and Price-Spratlen, T. (1999). Through the eyes of children: An ethnographic perspective on neighborhoods and child development. In A.S. Hasten (Ed.), *Cultural processes in child development* (pp. 77-96). Mahwah, NJ: Lawrence Erlbaum.

Coulton, C. (1996). The effects of neighborhoods on families and children: Implications for services. In A.J. Kahn and S.B. Kamerman (Eds.), *Children and their families in big cities* (pp. 87-120). New York: Columbia University School of Social Work Press.

Dixon, J. and Durrheim, K. (2000). Displacing place identity: A discursive approach to locating self and other. *British Journal of Social Psychology, 39*, 27-44.

Furstenberg, F. (1993). How families manage risk and opportunity in dangerous neighborhoods. In W. J. Wilson (Ed.), *Sociology and the public agenda* (pp. 231-258). Newbury Park, CA: Sage.

Garbarino, J., Galambos, N., Plantz, M., and Kostenly, K. (1992). The territory of childhood. In J. Garbarino (Ed.), *Children and families in the social environment,* Second edition (pp. 202-229). New York: Aldine de Gruyter.

Hart, R. (1979). *Children's experiences of place.* New York: Irvington.

Hart, R. (1997). *Children's participation: The theory and practice of involving young citizens in community development and environmental care.* London: Earthscan.

Kemp. S. (2001). Environment through a gendered lens: From person-in-environment to woman-in-environment. *Affilia, 16*(1), 7-30.

Lewis, M. and Osofsky, J. (1997). Violent cities, violent streets: Children draw their neighborhoods. In J. Osofsky (Ed.), *Children in a violent society* (pp. 277-299). New York: Guilford Press.

Moore, R. (1986). *Children's domain: Play and place in child development.* London: Croom Helm.

Nicotera, N. (in press). *Children and agency: The child's eye view of neighborhood change.* Unpublished manuscript.

Nicotera, N. (2003). Children and their neighborhoods: A mixed methods approach to understanding the construct neighborhood. *Dissertation Abstracts International* (UMI No. 3072123).

Perkins, D., Meeks, J., and Taylor, R. (1992). The physical environment of street blocks and residential perceptions of crime and disorder: Implications for theory and measurement. *Journal of Environmental Psychology, 12*, 21-34.

Sampson, R. and Raudenbush, S. (1999). Systematic social observation of public spaces: A new look at disorder in urban neighborhoods. *American Journal of Sociology, 105*(3), 603-651.

Schiavo, R.S. (1988). Age differences in assessment and use of a suburban neighborhood among children and adolescents. *Children's Environments Quarterly, 5*(2), 4-9.

Skejaeveland, O. and Garling, T. (1997). Effects of interactional space on neighboring. *Journal of Environmental Psychology, 17,* 181-198.

Sutton, S. (1992). Enabling children to map out a more equitable society. *Children's Environments, 9*(1), 37-48.

van Andel, J. (1990). Places children like, dislike, and fear. *Children's Environments Quarterly, 7*(4), 24-31.

Yuen, F. (2003). Critical concerns for family health practice. In F. Yuen, G. Skibinski, and J.T. Pardeck (Eds.), *Family health social work practice: A knowledge and skills casebook* (pp. 19-40). Binghamton, NY: The Haworth Social Work Practice Press.

Chapter 13

Family Health: Community Practice to Benefit Families and Children

John L. Erlich

INTRODUCTION

Humiliation. Perhaps more than any other single word, this captures the current state of health in poor communities across America. This suggests that the conditions of discrimination and oppression, despite massive political rhetoric to the contrary, have neither diminished nor disappeared. We welcome the media-celebrated ex-TANF (Temporary Assistance for Needy Families) mother getting a Harvard PhD, but her counterparts are few and far between. For most inner- city areas, as well as lower-income rural areas and suburbs, such stories seem a cruel joke. Somehow, apparently, with the proper attitude and hard work, anyone can make it big in America. This attitude is an important part of the reason that community-based efforts to support the health of children and families so often fall short of their goals. The minimal resources made available reflect this myth of hard work and positive attitude being all it takes for families to move out of poverty and racial segregation. Thus, by this backward reasoning, the person who cannot "make it" is only suffering the humiliation that she or he deserves.

BACKGROUND

How might we move beyond this self-limiting view of people living in communities with modest resources? In looking at community, Rothman (2001) suggests, "The community and its various elements provide the means for action and are the vehicle through which goals are achieved" (p. 11). Furthermore, Fellin (2001) notes, "The two sets of theory, human ecology and social systems, provide useful perspectives about spacial and geographic communities, as well as communities of identification and interest" (p. 119). This is not to suggest that other ways of looking at community, such as focusing on norms and values, studying history and leaders, and looking at unemployment and teen pregnancy data are not legitimate. Rather, it is to suggest that a framework of understanding that ignores patterns of influence and systems of power and control is doomed to inadequacy. However, part of the problem with a power-related analysis is that it is usually neither simple nor easily agreed upon. Indeed, as Carmichael and Hamilton (1967) noted during the Civil Rights Movement, "To define is to control." So it is that major battles continue to be fought over the definition of *community,* because communities are a major basis on which resources are allocated.

New York's Harlem-based Congressman Charles Rangel's proposal that the nation reimpose the draft not just to secure needed man- and womanpower for the military but also to make the playing field more level regarding the disproportionate numbers of poor and ethnic-minority young people carrying the burden in our military services, raised many eyebrows. The lack of response on both sides of the political aisle in Congress made it quite clear that most leading politicians wanted the idea to go away quietly.

Community History

If one really wants to have a sustainable impact on improving community health, there are a number of things that can be done. First, community history needs to be understood. As compared with people in many parts of the world, our personal sense of history in the United States tends to be very short range. It is almost as if we believe history is irrelevant because it will have little or no impact on what we do or how we do it. The pace of change appears to be so rapid as to render the past as a predictor of the future a minor factor. The past is not a minor factor by any means. Just as our ignorance and avoidance of history in Afghanistan and Iraq placed an enormous and unanticipated burden on our military, so too has our inability to take full account of community history and life led many well-meaning efforts in

America to founder because of lack of appreciation for why residents respond the way they do to overtures of "help."

From a broadly conceived standpoint of health, a number of areas may be considered useful, including history, employment, education, housing, institutions, libraries, and commerce.

Growth and Development Patterns

Among the important things to understand are the historical patterns of resident growth and development (especially in terms of immigrant and emigrant groups) within a community. Generational changes, particularly shifts in balance between first and second generations and second and third generations, require special attention (de Anda, 1997). The differences between generations (for example, the conflicts between first and second generation Vietnamese, Hmong, Mien, and Cambodians) are ignored at great peril to a community building effort. Varying Latino populations, especially among the more recent immigrants to the United States, often have similar intergenerational challenges. Illustratively, gender roles are often in transition in multigenerational and multiethnic communities (from male-dominated families and communities to more male-female equality, from early childbearing to later childbearing, etc.).

Employment

A second key area is that of employment. Patterns of work, both within and outside the community, are an important measure of people's sense of security and stability. Over time, what proportion of residents have been employed at a reasonable living wage? What proportion have of the population has health benefits?

When a particular commercial enterprise represents a significant proportion of employment in the community, it too should be viewed in the context of its changing and ongoing role in community life. For example, the potential hours of employment are not insignificant in relation to when and what time of day residents might be available to participate in what sort of activities.

Education

What about the schools? Clearly the quality of public education (and in some cases parochial education) as perceived by residents is another key factor in understanding their relative feelings of well-being. Again, over time has it gotten better, worse, or stayed about the same?

Housing

Housing is another vital arena. What is the extent of decent, safe housing in the community? How has the number of owners compared with renters been changing over time? Is there any significant increase in affordable housing for renters or owners in recent years? If not, why? Clearly this, too, measures health broadly conceived.

Institutions

In addition, a vital part of community history is often to be found in the development of its institutions, particularly its churches, mosques, and synagogues. The places in which people worship and exercise their faith, however we may personally view a particular religious observance, are often a useful guide to the strength of certain norms and values in subparts of almost all communities. Through their histories, the emergence and development of feelings toward new and emerging groups in the community (such as significant food and clothes closets) can often be tracked, as well as changing patterns of intergroup relations. Whether most of a congregation (or those in attendance) is local or from outside the area is instructive.

The role of the local public library (or libraries) can also be a useful piece of information. The more it sees itself as a community-based institution and less as a middle-class mission to the poor, the more likely it is to be a potential ally in local change efforts.

Community history and life can be gleaned from a variety of sources. Years ago, when I began my academic career, I was taken to lunch by a self-appointed mentor from the senior faculty. I ate my lunch. The mentor drank his. While this made for a somewhat uncomfortable atmosphere for digestion it also provided an opportunity to explore a broad spectrum of past institutional and community politics (especially old, unsettled grudges). Those who are somewhat marginal to the community, for example, an ex-leader of a voluntary community group can often provide useful "intelligence." Observed informal interactions among children, adolescents, and adults can be a useful gauge of community sentiment. Indeed, the informal interactions between different age groups, especially adolescents and adults, can be a vital indicator of areas of conflict and commonality.

Strengths, Resilience, and Empowerment

Although there are many perspectives from which appropriate family health practice at the community level may be viewed (for example, see Morrissey and Wandersman, 1995; Whittaker and Garbarino, 1983), for our purposes a strengths, resilience, and empowerment framework (Gutierrez, 1990) may be useful. As the nation's experience with the occupation of Iraq has made abundantly clear (in terms, for example, of not attending adequately to water supplies and waste disposal in the extreme heat of summer), inattention to basic needs can have disastrous consequences. In the absence of the necessary attention to essentials, support of existing community strengths and endurance becomes almost impossible. That is, community residents are likely to be very difficult to mobilize on their own behalf if they feel those in positions of power are determining *their* priorities. If a person is told he or she is worthy of directing his or her own affairs, and then is treated as if the belief is not true, a negative reaction can be expected.

Some areas of community health practice around which community people may be mobilized on their own behalf are as follows:

1. *Decent, safe housing:* Despite the very limited attention to housing at the national and state levels in the past decade, it is quite clear that this is a major issue in almost every poor, working-class, and inner-city community. Is there any construction of low and moderate income units? If so, are the amounts significant in relation to what is needed? If most housing is owned by absentee landlords, how widespread are code violations and maintenance problems? Do the residents feel a sense of pride in the way their community housing looks?

2. *Safe streets:* Are the streets safe? Are there places for children to play? For families to sit outside in the evening? Are lights and

stop signs adequate in comparison with more affluent nearby areas? Is the handling of garbage similar to that received in nearby affluent areas? What impact do drug traffic and gangs have on street safety?

3. *Adequate transportation:* To what degree is adequate public transportation (at a reasonable cost) available to the area? Does the pattern of public transportation suggest an assumption that most families will have their own (reliable) vehicles? Is the scheduling of public transportation responsive to community needs, especially in relation to work and child care?

4. *Day care:* Although the rhetoric emphasizes the importance of quality, affordable day care accompanying welfare-to-work programs, the reality is often very different. What are the day care options, what is the distance from most families' homes, and what is the cost (in relation to what most area families can afford)? Are appropriate subsidies readily available?

5. *Recreation:* The value and importance of physical exercise and activity has been well documented (Lappe, 1985). However, attention to the recreational needs of most communities tends to be focused on women and their preschool children, and on organized sports for teens and adults. This often results in elementary and middle-school students feeling neglected. Also, open spaces in many poor areas are dominated by older teens and young adults in ways that can make them somewhat unsafe places for young families and children alone.

Certainly there are many other important considerations in a reasonable assessment of health considerations at the community level. Some of these, such as HIV/AIDS and gangs, are addressed in other chapters in this text. Other considerations, such as levels of income, education, and infant mortality represent data typically collected and considered in community-health assessments. Here again, even a progressive public health perspective tends to reflect the priorities of health professionals rather than those of the people who live there.

COMMUNITY PRACTICE MODELS

We now turn to models for (1) assessing a community problem or issue and (2) developing a plan of action based on that assessment. It should be noted that there are many well-respected planning designs available (Lauffer, 1981), and the following design was selected largely on the basis of its clarity and directness. Profound, complex frameworks tend to be much more useful for intellectual conversation than to offer guidance for real-world intervention.

The designs noted here closely follow the work of Kirst-Ashman and Hull (2001). In some ways, the assessment of a problem or issue may be more important than the plan of action to address it in the sense that the way a problem or issue is considered (what is taken into account and what is not) has direct implications for the action that then might be taken. For example, the assessment of mental illness in a community may appear very different when based on the views of service providers than when based on the expressed concerns of community residents.

Let's briefly review each major component of the basic PREPARE design. A more elaborate and detailed illustration follows later in this chapter.

PROBLEMS. Identify problems you want to address.

REALITY. Review your community and personal reality.

ESTABLISH. Designate primary goals to achieve.

PEOPLE. Identify influential people.

ASSESS. Determine potential financial (and political) costs and benefits to clients and agency.

RISKS. Review professional and personal risks.

EVALUATE. Calculate the potential success of a community-change process.

Here, then, are guidelines for the IMAGINE plan of action, which builds from the assessment. Again, let's briefly review each major component.

IDEA. Begin with an innovative idea or action.

MUSTER. Formulate an action system and muster support.

ASSETS. Identify assets that may be mobilized.

GOALS. Identify goals, objectives, and action steps by which they may be attained.

IMPLEMENT the plan.

NEUTRALIZE opposition.

EVALUATE progress toward goals.

It might be noted that certain situations require a kind of direct action for which the models explored previously are not well adapted. Many of these are related to getting the attention of uninterested or reluctant powers-that-be in order for any significant change to occur. Traffic signs are a good, if modest, example. In many jurisdictions, getting a traffic light or even a stop sign for a corner at which there have been serious injuries or even deaths can be a process taking many months, if not years. However, a group of families blocking the intersection in question at rush hour may result in media attention that greatly speeds up the process.

Frequently, the focus of such mobilizations is how to make more equal the balance of power between community residents and political or economic institutions. Power, as Alinsky (1971) wisely noted, is not what you have but what the enemy thinks you have.

Many communities across the country have seen a rise in the numbers of homeless families (as distinguished from homeless single men and women) within the past years. The following illustration draws from the experiences of a number of cities in northern California. It clearly represents a very important aspect of our deteriorating community health. The PREPARE framework is used in the following.

1. *Problem(s):* The problem is this city is the increasing number of homeless families. In this case, with the exception of one very small, twelve-bed, church-sponsored facility limited to women and children, the city itself had no overnight shelters exclusively for families.
2. *Reality:* In this example we will develop the assessment from the perspective of someone already working in the city's main shelter. Her position enabled her to see the general view of overburdened, underfunded homeless services, a now old media story and unpopular service population, and more needy homeless people. Her personal knowledge of the population gave her both credibility with her human service colleagues and, at the same time, assigned her a role as a "bleeding heart" in the public mind. Her role also gave her some sense of the city's homeless "politics."
3. *Establish* (primary goals): The essential goal was the development of a substantial homeless shelter exclusively for women and children. Although a whole range of questions might be

asked about location, variety of services to be provided, staffing, etc., the primary objective was clear.

4. *People:* The key players identified were the mayor, the city council (especially those members who had supported shelters in the past), downtown business groups concerned about shelter impact on commerce, shelter providers, homeless advocates, the homeless themselves, and local newspaper columnists who had covered the homeless.

5. *Assess* (costs/benefits to agency and clients): Although resources could conceivably be taken from other shelter-related services to fund a family shelter, the potential benefits seem to far outweigh the costs (or risks). Certainly the current major shelter was unlikely to suffer any permanent damage in its community status because it was in no position to offer separate places for women and children in the existing, limited shelter complex. At the same time, the worker felt that dollars spent to serve women and children might be more easily obtained than to serve single men.

6. *Risks:* She also felt that her social work career would not be negatively impacted by her effort to secure shelter for families. It was her intention to let her superiors at the main shelter know what she was planning to do (indeed, it was her hope to enlist their support) so that any consequences for the main shelter might be considered.

7. *Evaluate* (potential success): Given the political climate of the time, and the general cutbacks in human service, the potential for success was regarded as moderate. Although women and children might be viewed as more "deserving" than single men (often men with substance abuse and/or mental health problems), they were not one of the more popular service populations.

Now explore an action plan based on the IMAGINE framework.

1. *Idea:* Basically, the worker's idea was to raise the level of awareness of the plight of homeless women and children in order to secure a family shelter. However, this was clearly easier said than done.

2. *Muster* (support and action): Here the worker had to make a critical judgment. Should she try to build the widest possible alliance of supportive groups and individuals, or instead, use the time and energy to put together a smaller but more vigorous group of activists, homeless advocates, and ex-homeless? She chose the latter.

3. *Assets:* The kind of assets to be mobilized were progressive women's organizations (including a local NOW [National Organization for Women] group); an alliance of churches providing volunteer services to the homeless; a homeless coalition consisting of people who had worked on the issue over the years, including ex-homeless; an outspoken minister who served on her shelter's board; and the two most liberal city council members. Preliminary contact would also be made with a newspaper reporter who had sympathetically covered the plight of the homeless in the past.

4. *Goals:* Her strategy included the following steps:
   • inviting a well-respected agency director of a day program serving the homeless and other street people to serve as a lead organizer for the coalition and temporary chairperson;
   • contacting individuals noted previously or whom the worker knew or had good reason to believe would strongly support the women's shelter idea as coalition members;
   • developing a statement of purpose in conjunction with the lead organizer focusing on documenting the urgent need for a family shelter;
   • setting up an initial meeting and inviting potential coalition members who had been previously contacted to confirm their interest in participating;
   • preparing the agenda for the meeting and a draft statement that, in final agreed-upon revision, could be presented to the media as well as to the appropriate political bodies; and
   • asking for a commitment (launched by the two most liberal city council members) to study the question for no more than three months before returning to the council and other appropriate funding sources with a recommendation.

5. *Implement:* This plan, similar to most plans, did not go precisely as outlined, although it did come pretty close. Most problems were due to the worker having to chair the initial meeting because the lead organizer was twenty-five minutes late, and hav-

ing a reporter not show up for an interview. The city council members, rather than having their staff study the plan, decided to ask three organizations currently serving the homeless in some fashion (along with others who were interested) to submit detailed proposals in ninety days.

6. *Neutralize* (opposition): Although the effort did not mobilize a large amount of community support, it also did not generate strong, concerted opposition. The church leaders in the coalition offered to speak to interested or concerned churches and business groups. The statement of purpose made it clear that taking resources from existing homeless services to provide a shelter for women and children would not be acceptable. Public support was generated around the appropriate meetings of the city council rather than being aimed at a broader public (such as the timing of press releases, and accepting interview offers from columnists rather than big story reporters).

7. *Evaluate* (progress): With the staff support of the shelter worker, the lead organizer (and coalition chair), along with the now-named Family Shelter Task Force that received periodic reports, the shelter worker kept tabs on progress toward the ultimate objective of establishing a family shelter. Eight months from the first meeting it became a reality. Although the road from humiliation to participation and empowerment is neither clearly defined nor easy, there are some guideposts and steps along the way for community health practice. The next move is up to the reader.

DISCUSSION QUESTIONS, EXERCISES, AND RECOMMENDED READINGS

Discussion Questions

The questions below are intended to help the reader explore, in more personal and professional detail, aspects of the major service areas addressed in this chapter. The questions are not intended to suggest that they are either the most important or that they cover anywhere near the full range of appropriate questions. Hopefully, they are at least a place to start.

1. What sort of a place is the community in which you grew up? (Such areas as the mix and relative proportions of racial, ethnic, and religious groups; kinds and cost of housing; public transportation; larger businesses and commercial enterprises; educational and recreational opportunities, etc.)
2. What sort of place is the community in which you currently live?
3. What are the most urgent community health problems? (A broad perspective is recommended here, including such factors as unemployment, homelessness, street safety, underperforming, schools, exploitation of undocumented workers, and the adequacy of culturally competent mental health services to serving those with HIV/AIDS.)
4. Who is involved in public discussions about these problems and issues? (Such community actors as local politicians, community leaders and organizations, service providers, community residents, and college-based activists might be considered.)
5. Has there been a significant change in those discussions in the past two or three years in terms of leadership and influence? Or within whatever time frame you have had a chance to observe them? (Here the intention is to especially consider the patterns of who is more and less influential over time, and in relation to what issues. If known, the formation of alliances and coalitions should not be neglected.)
6. Who gets credit when progress is made in dealing with these problems and and issues? (Particularly the balance between credit given to political figures and institutional leaders as compared with community-based people might be addressed here.)
7. Who gets blamed when things go badly in dealing with these problems and issues? (Here, too, a primary recommended focus is the balance of blame received by politicians and institutional leaders as compared with community people.)
8. What community agencies or organizations have the most potential to have a significant impact on these problems and issues? (This is part of the search for leaders and allies in the change process.)
9. Where plans are going forward to address these problems and issues, what provisions are being made to involve community people on their own behalf? Assume leadership roles?

Exercises

Here are a couple of possible classroom exercises that may be used to explore the community-health perspectives developed in this chapter.

Depending on the size of the class, break up into three to six small groups (probably no more than six or seven students in each) to explore a problem/issue such as teen pregnancy. Each group can be charged to first arrive at a consensus on the nature of the problem (teen girls, boys/men, parental supervision, morals and values, availability of birth control information and devices, the schools, media, etc.) and then, using the IMAGINE framework (some parts of PREPARE may be useful as well), develop a simple basic plan of action and present it to the class. Perhaps a minimum of three to four hours should be allotted for discussion and preparation, and twenty to thirty minutes for each group to present to the whole class. Variants of this include having half of the groups deal with one topic, and the other half another (such as street violence), or each group being assigned a different topic.

Another approach is to have the class select topics (numbers of topics based on group assignments), which are then assigned randomly to the groups.

In the initial stages it is important that ample class time be allotted for preliminary discussions so that assistance can be provided if groups run into trouble establishing basic frameworks or guidelines for action plan development.

Recommended Readings

A variety of broader and more in-depth perspectives are to be found in the readings listed below.

Alinsky, S. (1971). *Rules for radicals*. New York: Vintage Books.

Austin, M. J. and Lowe, J. I. (1994). *Controversial issues in communities and organizations*. Needham Heights, MA: Allyn & Bacon.

Burghardt, S. (1982). *Organizing for community action*. Beverly Hills: Sage.

Erlich, J., Rothman, J., and Teresa, J. (1999). *Taking action in organizations and communities*. Dubuque, IA: Eddie Bowers.

Homan, M. (1999). *Promoting community change: Making it happen*, Second edition. Pacific Grove, CA: Brooks/Cole.

Kirst-Ashman, J. and Hull, G. (1999). *Understanding generalist practice*, Second edition. Chicago: Nelson Hall.
Kirst-Ashman, J. and Hull, G. (2001). *Generalist practice with organizations and communities*, Second edition. Belmont, CA: Wadsworth.
Rivera, F. and Erlich, J. (1998). *Community organizing in a diverse society*, Third edition. Needham, MA: Allyn & Bacon.
Tropman, J., Erlich, J., and Rothman, J. (2001). *Tactics and techniques of community intervention*, Fourth edition. Itasca, IL: F. E. Peacock
Weil, M. and Gamble, D. (1995). Community Practice Models. In *Encyclopedia of social work*, Nineteenth edition, Volume 1 (pp. 577-593). Washington, DC: NASW Press.

REFERENCES

Alinsky, S. (1971). *Rules for radicals*. New York: Vintage Books.
Carmichael, S. and Hamilton, C. (1967). *Black power: The politics of liberation in America*. New York: Vintage.
de Anda, D. (1997). *Controversial issues in multiculturalism*. Needham, MA: Allyn & Bacon.
Fellin, P. (2001). Understanding American communities. In J. Rothman, J. Erlich, and J. Tropman (Eds.), *Strategies of community intervention*, Sixth edition (pp. 114-129). Itasca, IL: F. E. Peacock.
Gutierrez, L. (1990). Working with women of color: An empowerment perspective. *Social Work*, 35, 149-153.
Kirst-Ashman, K. and Hull, G. (2001). *Generalist practice with organizations and communities*, Second edition. Belmont, CA.: Wadsworth.
Lappe, F. (1985). *What to do after you turn off the T.V.: Fresh ideas for enjoying family time*. New York: Ballantine.
Lauffer, A. (1981). The practice of social planning. In N. Gilbert and H. Specht (Eds.), *Handbook of the social services*. Englewood Cliffs, NJ: Prentice Hall.
Morrissey, E. and Wandersman, A. (1995). Total quality management in health care settings: A preliminary framework for successful implementation. In L. Ginsberg and P. Keys (Eds.), *New Management in Human Services*, Second edition, (pp. 171-194). Washington, DC: NASW Press.
Rothman, J. (2001). Introduction. In J. Rothman, J. Erlich, and J. Tropman (Eds.), *Strategies of community intervention*, Sixth edition (pp. 3-26). Itasca, IL: F. E. Peacock.
Whittaker, J. and Garbarino, J. (1983). *Social support networks: Informal helping in the human services*. New York: Aldine.

Index

Page numbers followed by the letter "b" indicate boxed text; those followed by the letter "f" indicate figures; and those followed by the letter "t" indicate tables.

Order a copy of this book with this form or online at:
http://www.haworthpress.com/store/product.asp?sku=5305

SOCIAL WORK PRACTICE WITH CHILDREN AND FAMILIES
A Family Health Approach

_____in hardbound at $39.95 (ISBN: 0-7890-1795-4)

_____in softbound at $24.95 (ISBN: 0-7890-1796-2)

Or order online and use special offer code HEC25 in the shopping cart.

COST OF BOOKS_____

☐ **BILL ME LATER:** (Bill-me option is good on US/Canada/Mexico orders only; not good to jobbers, wholesalers, or subscription agencies.)

☐ Check here if billing address is different from shipping address and attach purchase order and billing address information.

POSTAGE & HANDLING_____
(US: $4.00 for first book & $1.50 for each additional book)
(Outside US: $5.00 for first book & $2.00 for each additional book)

Signature_____

SUBTOTAL_____

☐ **PAYMENT ENCLOSED:** $_____

IN CANADA: ADD 7% GST_____

☐ **PLEASE CHARGE TO MY CREDIT CARD.**

STATE TAX_____
(NJ, NY, OH, MN, CA, IL, IN, & SD residents, add appropriate local sales tax)

☐ Visa ☐ MasterCard ☐ AmEx ☐ Discover
☐ Diner's Club ☐ Eurocard ☐ JCB

Account # _____

FINAL TOTAL_____
(If paying in Canadian funds, convert using the current exchange rate. UNESCO coupons welcome)

Exp. Date_____

Signature_____

Prices in US dollars and subject to change without notice.

NAME_____

INSTITUTION_____

ADDRESS_____

CITY_____

STATE/ZIP_____

COUNTRY_____ COUNTY (NY residents only)_____

TEL_____ FAX_____

E-MAIL_____

May we use your e-mail address for confirmations and other types of information? ☐ Yes ☐ No
We appreciate receiving your e-mail address and fax number. Haworth would like to e-mail or fax special discount offers to you, as a preferred customer. **We will never share, rent, or exchange your e-mail address or fax number.** We regard such actions as an invasion of your privacy.

Order From Your Local Bookstore or Directly From
The Haworth Press, Inc.
10 Alice Street, Binghamton, New York 13904-1580 • USA
TELEPHONE: 1-800-HAWORTH (1-800-429-6784) / Outside US/Canada: (607) 722-5857
FAX: 1-800-895-0582 / Outside US/Canada: (607) 771-0012
E-mailto: orders@haworthpress.com

For orders outside US and Canada, you may wish to order through your local
sales representative, distributor, or bookseller.
For information, see http://haworthpress.com/distributors

(Discounts are available for individual orders in US and Canada only, not booksellers/distributors.)
PLEASE PHOTOCOPY THIS FORM FOR YOUR PERSONAL USE.
http://www.HaworthPress.com   BOF04